AF179647

UNDERSTANDING AND MANAGING DEMENTIA

Joan C. Breitung, RN, MA, MSN

ISBN: 09707558 4 8

North American Address:
5840 Corporate Way, Suite 200, West Palm Beach, FL 33407
Tel: (561) 697-1447

European Address:
50 Highpoint, Heath Road, Weybridge, Surrey KT13 8TP, UK
Tel: (44) (0) 1932 844526, Fax: (44) (0) 1932 820419

E-mail: garevpub@aol.com

TABLE OF CONTENTS

TABLE OF CONTENTS cont.

INTRODUCTION

The term dementia describes a group of symptoms that are caused by changes in brain function. These symptoms affect thinking, learning and memory abilities. For example, those who are affected become lost in familiar places, are unable to follow directions, become disoriented about time, people, and places and neglect their personal safety, hygiene, and nutrition.

Governments in developed countries are presently dealing with the enormous strain on public services caused by the devastating effects of dementia. However, awareness of this disorder is just beginning to emerge in developing countries. Sixty six percent of people with dementia live in developing countries and the numbers are increasing, particularly in the heavily populated regions of China, India and Latin America.

Dementing disorders can surface rapidly, as in the case of brain injury, or slowly and insidiously as happens with Alzheimer's disease. Day by day dementia steadily robs an individual of independence and dignity. Patients and their caregivers constantly face situations ranging from the unpleasant to the unimaginable as life's routine daily activities progressively become huge health and safety issues. Daily life becomes turbulent because major decisions regarding finances, medication regimens, creating a living will, designating a health care proxy or arranging an alternative living situation must be made promptly. Consequently, in addition to the imposition of time and financial constraints, caregivers bear very high levels of emotional and physical strain. Sometimes it is a frail elderly spouse who assumes this responsibility, but more often an adult child is thrust into the situation, equally ill-prepared to manage the burden of the disorder.

Alzheimer's disease and related dementias exact a massive toll in health care costs, disability, and lost productivity of both patients and family caregivers. Although most of the people with dementia are retired and are not losing income because of their disease, the cost of their care is still prohibitive. By most estimates, the global issue of dementia costs hundreds of billions in dollars in lost annual productivity and direct care costs, exclusive of the care provided by family caregivers. Global figures include:

- One in 10 persons over 65 years of age and nearly half of those over 85 years old have Alzheimer's disease.
- A small percentage of people in their 30s and 40s get the disease.
- 12 million individuals worldwide, have Alzheimer's disease. By 2025, that number will increase to 22 million.
- Although more than four million Americans are afflicted with Alzheimer's disease, millions more have other reversible or irreversible dementias.

- There are approximately 6 million sufferers in the European Union and 800,000 in the UK.
- In Canada, more than 300,000 people have Alzheimer's disease. By 2031, the number will increase to 750,000.

Many of today's 'baby boomers'- those born between 1942 and 1964 - are finding themselves in the exhausting and bewildering role of caregiver for a disabled parent while working and caring for their own families. However, these figures will soar when those baby boomers reach old age.

Dementia is the reason for more than half of all nursing home admissions. It is a major public health problem that affects everyone in terms of morbidity, mortality, quality of life issues and health care costs. Nevertheless, early detection of dementia before an individual becomes severely impaired has several potential benefits:

- Reversible causes of dementia can be identified and treated.
- Therapy to slow the progression of disease can be initiated.
- Steps can be taken to reduce the morbidity (illnesses) associated with dementia.
- Patients and their families can prepare for problems that will surface as dementia progresses.

Although there are medications and therapies that clinicians have to offer, there are still too many undiagnosed cases, untreated patients and families in despair.

Understanding And Managing Dementia describes the disorders, lists potential causes and treatment options, and addresses timely issues for clinicians, health care administrators, policy makers and educators. Caregivers, especially, will use this worthwhile resource when asessing their own strengths and limitations. It can empower them to effectively manage their responsibilities by using appropriate behavioral strategies, treatment options and health care agencies.

The increasingly dependent state of patients with dementia alters relationships and often overwhelms caregivers. Studies have shown that dementia caregivers experience higher levels of stress and depression than do caregivers for terminally ill cancer patients. This is because they have to contend with so many unforeseen and atypical behavioral problems their loved ones develop such as wandering, verbal aggression, or destruction of property. Another contributing factor to the greater pressure experienced by the caregiver may also be the anticipation that not only will things get worse, but that this will surely happen in an unpredictable and uncontrollable manner.

Becoming informed and maximizing the use of the available resources provide caregivers with a measure of control. It also helps them to respond constructively when dealing with a family member who is inevitably and profoundly changed by a dementing illness.

Joan C. Breitung

CHAPTER 1

Aging and Memory Impairment

Few disorders are dreaded more by older adults and their families than dementia, the disability that destroys minds, ruins relationships and can cause the death of the patient. This fear is not groundless. The World Health Organization estimates that the total number of people worldwide that are affected by the various forms of dementia has reached more than 29 million. Global population aging inevitably will result in huge increases in the number of cases of dementia and the risks rise sharply in adults over 60.

By 2020 the world population aged 60 years and older will exceed one billion, with more than 700 million living in developing countries. By the year 2025, those with dementia may surpass 80 million in Africa, Asia, and Latin America alone. Globally, dementia can afflict a staggering 25 percent in some of the oldest age groups. Since aging intensifies the range of mental health issues, the aging world population is a pressing, fundamental development issue that demands the attention of world leaders and policy makers in addition to every health care professional.

Powerful social, personal and financial impacts are reflected in global estimates. As an example, the financial burden of dementia, including direct care costs and lost productivity, is projected to be in the 100s of billions of dollars annually, an assessment that excludes the cost of direct care by family caregivers.

The term dementia is widely recognized as signifying certain losses of intellectual function, chiefly memory, language, and judgment as well as many related behavioral aberrations. When dementia is mentioned, the first thought that usually comes to mind is Alzheimer's disease (AD). This is a natural response because Alzheimer's disease is well known and accounts for more than half of the dementias. Although other dementing disorders may be less familiar, they are no less devastating in their effects on families and their stricken loved ones.

Stereotypes of old age

Families and clinicians may attribute some of the early signs of dementing illnesses to a stereotypical view of old age as the following case study illustrates:

A woman who lived several hundred miles away from her parents recently confided that she received an alarming phone call from her parents' neighbor. The neighbor told her that her mother was driving erratically, seldom recognized her, and could not remember how to run the washing machine in the senior housing complex where they lived. She immediately called her father and asked him to explain her mother's behavior, but all he did was deny that anything was wrong and accused the neighbor of meddling. She then bought a plane ticket and was preparing to leave in order to find out for herself just how serious things were. " I guess it's senility," she said sadly, "something I should have expected since they're both in their 70's now."

Senility is a loose, poorly defined term that once was applied to any diminished mental function experienced by an older adult. Although normal aging is characterized by slower recall of information and a longer processing time for new data, neither alteration is an indication of 'senility'. Nevertheless, many elderly wrongly bear this label. It is one of the many myths of aging and a prejudice that older adults must reluctantly endure.

The assumption that once a person reaches the age of 65, certain intellectual functions such as thinking, remembering, and decision-making will gradually deteriorate, can have dangerous consequences. If such changes do occur and families regard them as part of the normal aging process, much the same as one expects to see elderly persons with gray hair and wrinkled skin, medical intervention may be delayed and valuable time is lost.

It is not a myth, however, to claim that the aging process affects the brain just as it does the rest of the body. New imaging technology clearly shows that with aging brain tissue thins and as a result there is some brain shrinkage with aging, but exactly how these changes affects its multi-tasking operation is still unclear.

Overall, the changes are not as devastating as once reported. For example, brain cells are not lost in the large numbers that was once thought and there is evidence to support the claim that in certain situations even an old brain is capable of producing new cells.

The brain is composed of billions of nerve cells called neurons that are in constant communication with each other transmitting life-sustaining information that enables the body to exist and operate to full capacity. All the complexities of each physical, mental, and emotional function are either voluntarily or involuntarily governed by the brain. To illustrate: whether a person is savoring a meal (involuntary) or running in a race (voluntary) both activities involve intricate physical and chemical signals and processes that originate in the brain. It is only when a significant malfunction occurs that anyone would be aware of a problem.

If asked, most older adults would probably admit that they are concerned about becoming forgetful. However, not all memory problems are serious. It is far more common to learn of older adults who remain both alert and competent throughout their lifespans, although most of them would concur that recalling information takes somewhat longer than it used to. On the other hand, there are times when memory problems are the earliest indication of a brain dysfunction. For example, almost everyone has been annoyed at one time or another by misplacing his or her keys. This is a commonplace, everyday experience. However, when an elderly person cannot recall what keys are used for, that may be a significant sign of dementia.

The onset of cognitive impairment is insidious because it occurs so slowly that it is barely noticeable. The early episodes of poor memory experienced by the dementia patient are generally met either with denial or explained away as just a case of absentmindedness or, more likely, stress. But the ready excuses for the changes in behavior and mood inevitably disappear as the dementia advances. In addition to memory impairment, the other common markers of dementia are: repeatedly asking the same questions, increased irritability, the disappearance of social skills, indifference to hygiene and the inability for self care. Eventually someone in the family is forced to admit that medical help is needed.

CASE STUDY

Alma, an 85-year-old widow, lives alone in the same neighborhood she moved to as a bride. There were many changes over the years, but Alma was always comfortable in her small apartment and she saw no reason to move. The supermarket was just a few blocks away and she easily managed the walk to church and her hairdresser's for punctual, weekly visits.

Alma enjoyed frequent visits from her son, who lived nearby. Then, abruptly, he was transferred to another state and for almost four months he did not see his mother. Rather, he depended on frequent phone calls to keep in touch. Slowly, though, he began to develop uneasy feelings after those calls. Although she denied that anything was wrong, his mother's voice was toneless when she spoke to him and she always seemed distracted.

On impulse one week-end, he stopped in and surprised her. When she opened the door he was shocked. Alma wore a soiled bathrobe and her hair hung in greasy tangles. A foul odor in the apartment emanated from the kitchen where he saw the table and the sink covered with unopened mail and dirty dishes. Peering into the refrigerator he found only a container of spoiled milk and some moldy cheese; in the freezer were nine identical frozen dinners. Alma's formerly well stocked cupboard held three boxes of cereal and a few teabags.

When she was seen by a physician, Alma could tell him who she was, but that was about all. She was unable to answer his other questions and she did not understand a few simple commands such as "put the book on the chair" and "close your eyes". More important, she failed to identify some ordinary household items namely, a clock and a spoon.

The previous story is an example of an elderly lady who appears to have advancing dementia. In just a few months Alma went from carrying on a normal conversation to being unable to answer correctly questions about the current year, season and month. She was unable to follow simple commands or to identify common household objects. These developments indicated a distinct cognitive decline.

In many cases this damage is reversible. If Alma's dementia was caused by the side effects of a medication, an infection, or dehydration, it might be readily corrected with standard treatment. It is also possible that Alma's symptoms were caused by depression, the most common mental health disorder seen in the elderly, and which accurately mimics dementia. One thing is certain: her disorder is not caused by old age.

Symptoms of cognitive decline are not a normal part of the aging process, and no one should assume that it is. Eventually, a careful review of the lady's medications revealed that confusion and fatigue were frequent side effects of two of her drugs. She was also severely dehydrated and mildly depressed. This patient responded well to treatment for her dehydration and mild depression after her drug regimen was modified.

Influence of lifestyle

Although everyone feels threatened by the possibility of declining mental functioning, any idea that modern culture may have of aging being linked to mental incompetence is steadily being refuted by science and by the activities of most older adults. There are countless studies of elderly individuals with energetic lifestyles that are enhanced by exercise and healthful eating. These carefully researched groups have repeatedly demonstrated unimpaired intellectual functioning. However, these are the same older adults who took advantage of every available health maintenance opportunity, such as getting their immunizations for influenza and pneumonia, controlling their blood pressure, and challenging their brains with activities of new learning or with cards or board games.

Ageism

The brain is the source of many exacting functions such as the ability to analyze what is perceived through the five senses, to concentrate and make decisions, to interpret language, and to perform voluntary and involuntary movements. Normally, these actions are taken for granted until some mental or physical problem causes a malfunction.

Historically, confusion and memory loss were considered to be a corollary of growing older. Many people still mistakenly believe that mental disorders like depression and dementia are normal in older people and that no effective treatments are available. Another myth suggests that older adults cannot change, experience psychological and spiritual growth, or contribute to society. Therefore, efforts to enhance their mental health are futile.

There are still some health professionals and older adults who are quick to attribute memory and behavior abnormalities to aging, although fortunately their numbers are diminishing. The last decade has been one of accelerated research in the fields of the neurological and behavioral sciences. As a result, what was formerly unknown about the most complex organ in the body, the brain, is now better understood.

The old, negative stereotypes of aging are under scrutiny. It takes time to eradicate ageist prejudices but inevitably the hordes of adults presently in their 50s and early 60s will help to dispel forever the idea that to be old means to be cognitively impaired.

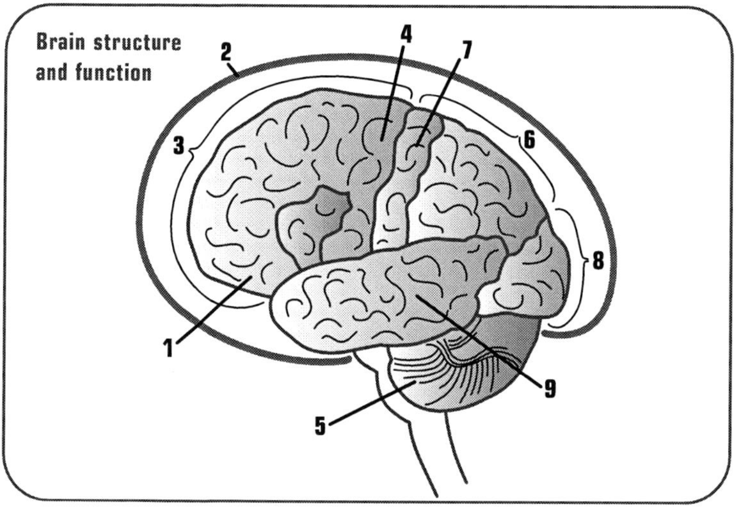

Figure 1.1 The Brain

Structure	Function
1. cerebellum	controls coordination of fine voluntary muscle movement i.e. writing, playing musical instruments
2. cerebrum	interprets sensory stimulation; center of memory, learning, judgment
3. frontal lobes	contributes to ability to plan and reason
4. motor areas	help to control voluntary movement
5. Broca's area	converts thoughts into words
6.&7. parietal lobes	primary sensory areas; processes information about taste, smell, touch, temperature and movement; governs reading and math skills
8. occipital lobes	processes images from the eyes and coordinates the information with images stored in memory
9. temporal lobes	processes auditory information; plays essential part in forming and retrieving memories including those associated with music; thought to integrate memories and sensations of taste, sound, touch.

Table 1.1 structure and function of areas of the brain.
Source: Institute of Neurologic Disorders and Stroke, National Institutes of Health. www.ninds.nih.gov/index

Under normal circumstances, few people think about any parts of the brain much less the complex operations it performs. As an example, when an individual tastes a favorite food, there is no thought given to which part of the brain governs this function. The food is simply tasted and enjoyed. Nonetheless, even a rudimentary understanding of the interdependence of each area of the brain is a sobering reminder of the scope of its multiple functions.

The illustration of the brain, the three pound organ housed within the skull, and its multipurpose regions highlights a few of the many activities that occur automatically, continually, and without an individual's awareness. However, when even a small area of the brain tissue is damaged, the effects can be immediate and catastrophic. Injuries that appear to be benign can quickly result in a major physical or mental impairment.

Disorders confused with dementia

As mentioned earlier, some of the signs of dementia are easily confused with other well known mind-altering disorders. For example, short-term memory loss, confusion, and inappropriate or bizarre behavior are also symptoms of the medical disorders of delirium, depression, and psychosis. All three of these disorders cause major alterations in a person' s memory and cognition, yet none of them is dementia.

Disorder	Symptoms	Cause
Delirium: an alteration in consciousness with a sudden onset of acute but temporary confusion.	Anxiety, disorientation, tremors, hallucinations, delusions, incoherence	Drug toxicity, alcoholism, malnutrition, heart/lung diseases, infections, hormonal disorders
Depression: a mood disorder characterized by despondency; common in older adults.	Sadness, apathy, difficulty in thinking and concentrating; feelings of despair. Changes in sleep patterns and appetite	May be related to chronic physical problems.
Psychosis: a mental disorder characterized by loss of contact with reality.	Delusions, hallucinations, paranoia.	Chronic alcoholism, drug ingestion, chemical imbalance.

Table 1.2 disorders which alter mental status.

delirium

Individuals with delirium are regularly seen in hospitals and long- term care settings. This acute confused state is generally triggered when a person has more than one illness - a typical occurrence in an older adult. Delirium develops in a matter of hours and manifests itself as a sudden case of confusion. A hypertensive patient who is admitted with a fractured hip is at a high risk for developing delirium because of the side effects of the medications prescribed concomitantly for high blood pressure and a hip fracture.

The active ingredient of many popular over-the-counter antihistamines and sleep aids is diphenhydramine. Known side effects of such drugs are drowsiness and, to a degree, confusion. Furthermore, diphenhydramine must also be used with great caution by anyone with thyroid disease, heart disease, high blood pressure or diabetes. If ingested in combination with alcohol or other drugs, adverse effects can rise to dangerous levels. Diphenhydramine has been linked to the increased risk of delirium as well as disorganized speech, and the inability to concentrate.

However, the opportunity for delirium to develop is not limited to drug reactions. Other causes of delirium are the onset of infections and the experience of being in an acute care setting. Older adults are profoundly affected by the disruptive occurrence of being admitted to a hospital and then being subjected to all its unfamiliar routines.

Delirium is a serious disorder and it is a reminder to all health care professionals that every hospitalization of an elderly person is a high-risk event.

depression

Depression (see Chapter 2.) is the most common mental health disorder affecting elderly individuals. Depression is often mistaken for dementia since some of its symptoms, e.g., memory loss, difficulty in concentrating, sad expression, and melancholy mood are similar to those seen in older adults with dementia. Anxiety often compounds the problems of untreated, depressed geriatric patients. Experienced health care workers in hospitals and nursing homes can testify to numerous incidents of elderly patients who displayed destructive behaviors by pulling out catheters and IV's, tearing off dressings, and refusing their medications. All of these actions are typical behaviors seen in geriatric patients who are depressed.

There is reason to be optimistic about depression, however. When the malady is correctly identified, it can be effectively treated. Successful treatment, however, depends to a large extent on the attitudes and cooperation of patients, family members, and clinicians. Two of the many popular and widely held misconceptions about the disorder of depression are, 1) it will eventually go away of its own accord and 2) old people cannot be treated successfully. Both views are false. When the older adult has appropriate medical management even the most seriously depressed person can be helped.

psychosis

Psychotic disorders, whether primary or secondary, are among the most serious psychiatric illnesses at any age. As the life expectancy continues to rise, however, health care systems will be severely strained trying to meet the needs of a disproportionate number of elderly psychotic patients.

These pressures will inevitably develop since psychosis is directly related to increases in the risks of institutionalization, mortality, and public expense.

Schizophrenia is a primary psychotic disorder and it can occur as late-onset or early-onset. Regardless of when the disease begins, the latest research yields evidence that it is much more common than previously believed. Psychosis also exists secondarily in certain medical conditions, e.g., substance abuse, Parkinson's disease and Alzheimer's disease. The most common form of secondary psychosis is found in patients with Alzheimer's disease.

Polypharmacy can contribute to psychotic symptoms. This possibility must always be considered since older adults consume more medication than any other age group and sustain up to three times as many adverse reactions from drugs.

It is important to note that the psychotic features of auditory and visual hallucinations or paranoid delusions are seen in a large number of Alzheimer's patients. The prevalence of agitation is seen in 75 to 90 percent of all nursing home patients at some point whether or not they have AD. Practical treatment goals for the elderly psychotic are targeted towards the relief of symptoms and the improvement in the ability to perform the activities of daily life.

Diagnosing dementia

Dementia is easy to recognize when it is advanced and the patient is profoundly disabled. However, it can be very difficult to diagnose when it is in the early stages. It is during this critical period that patients, families, and clinicians may underestimate the initial symptoms and mistakenly attribute them to the consequences of aging. Despite the extensive occurrence of dementia in older adults it is a disorder that is still frequently overlooked or misdiagnosed.

When someone in the family finally concludes that a memory problem is serious enough to be investigated, the first appointment is generally with a primary care physician. This appointment will be longer than a routine visit to a doctor. In addition to the usual patient history and physical examination the clinician will require a complete blood screening, tests of the liver and thyroid function, and whatever imaging technologies deemed useful to help confirm a diagnosis. The following are examples of scans used in such evaluations:

- computerized tomography (CT)
- magnetic resonance imaging (MRI)
- single photon emission tomography (SPECT)
- positron emission tomography (PET)

Part of the patient evaluation will be an examination by a neurologist and a psychiatrist. The relationship between patient and doctor is a sensitive one so it is important that the older adult understands that the role of any family member is mainly that of support and reassurance. The doctor will first see the patient alone, and then later invite the relative to be present – providing that the patient consents. It is advisable that the primary caregiver communicates clearly from the beginning a desire to be an active part of the patient's health care team.

A mental status examination is another important tool with which to assess a patient's thinking, emotional functioning and behavior. Essentially, the physician will question the individual about his orientation to person, place and time. The testing includes repeating words, doing simple math problems and drawing figures. During this time the answers are evaluated as well as the way patient responds verbally and his general behavior.

A study published in the Archives of Neurology, December, 2003, compared the Mini-Mental Status Examination (MMSE) and the Short Test of Mental Status. The conclusion was that the Short Test of Mental Status was better able to confirm mild cognitive impairment (MCI), a harbinger of Alzheimer's disease. Moreover, it was more sensitive in detecting deficits in cognition in individuals who had normal awareness and insight at baseline but later developed MCI or AD.

Clinicians and consumers need to bear in mind, however, that no test can be used alone to diagnose dementia. Clinical judgment and extensive neuropsychological testing are other important components of the process.

(For an example of a mental status examination, please see appendix 4.)

How caregivers can help with treatment

Treating dementia involves much more than simply prescribing the right medication. It may also require lifestyle changes such a diet and exercise plan as well as the modification of any other factors that can improve health. Caregivers who are adult children or spouses, need to understand and support the physician's treatment strategy. When patients or their caregivers do not fully grasp the meaning of the medical condition or the plan for treatment, there is little chance for either compliance or success. Not knowing what is wrong is discouraging to both the patients and their families, so it is vital to ask questions and clear up any misunderstandings.

If the diagnosis confirms that the dementia is irreversible, questions often arise about disclosure. The main question is, is it appropriate to tell the patient his disease will progress? The answer depends on what the patient wants to know and how well his mind is working at the time. There are many benefits to receiving the diagnosis early in the disease. Two of the more pressing arguments for early diagnosis are for financial and legal planning, such as making a will and selecting an executor, and for preparing a healthcare proxy and a living will.

Most adults who have reached late life have worked very hard to accumulate and maintain an estate. The best way to ensure that someone's wishes are carried out and to maintain harmony within the family is take advantage of professional advice and to do so in a timely manner.

A living will is a document that specifies a person's preference for medical care if they are incapacitated. A durable power of attorney is a document in which someone (the proxy) is empowered to make medical decisions for the person who is unable to do so.

Determining what kind of medical intervention an individual will either permit or refuse when an illness reaches a terminal state is a very serious decision, and naming a proxy to make healthcare decisions for another individual is an equally grave judgment. Often the pressures of clinical emergencies may override one's wishes. Clearly, the preferred time to make these weighty decisions is when individuals and their families are able to learn and evaluate their choices.

Since both of these documents are created before they are used they are called 'advance directives'. Advance directive laws vary from state to state as well as among locations abroad, but standard forms can generally be obtained from hospitals, medical associations, departments of elder affairs, or various community agencies that assist the elderly. Creating these documents may be the most important decisions the patient will ever have to make and if done in the early stages of a disease, there is great satisfaction and peace of mind in having exercised this control.

Patients and families also need to be aware of some of the other advantages of receiving an early diagnosis:

- expensive and inappropriate treatment can be avoided
- practical therapies can be developed to manage certain symptoms such as depression, wandering, and incontinence
- investigations can be made about acquiring more help at home or exploring the aspects of residential care

There is no denying that the diagnosis of an irreversible dementia is extremely sad and distressing to receive, but it is unlikely that the disorder will advance rapidly. Patients and their families usually will have some time to adapt. During this time there is still much that a caregiver can do to enhance and improve the patient's quality of life.

An initial priority will be to ensure the safety of both caregiver and patient. Daily routines can be modified and the environment in the home can be adapted. The whole family can participate in helping to create a safe, secure home environment.

CASE STUDY

Emma recently moved her 79-year-old mother out of an assisted living setting and brought her home. Her mother was diagnosed with Parkinson's disease and Emma was determined to care for her.

After spending many hours reading about safety precautions, she worked very hard to modify her home. She removed the scatter rugs, installed grab bars in the bathroom, improved the lighting and checked the batteries in each smoke detector. She even remembered to lower the temperature of the hot water. The only thing she overlooked was the possibility that her mother might wander. She was caught off guard when one day her mother simply walked out of the house. After frantically searching the neighborhood the first few times her mother disappeared, she remembered that the drycleaning shop had a buzzer, which sounded as each customer opened the door. Emma lost no time having sensors installed on all doors. Although her mother still tried to leave the house, a sensor would sound and alert Emma or her daycare worker so that one of them could intercept the patient.

Caregivers can learn to anticipate the elderly person's needs for comfort and safety before facing a crisis situation. There are extensive community resources, local support groups and expert advice available from governmental agencies. As they plan safety measures, families need to expect that emergency situations will arise. In order to save time and minimize worry it is helpful to prominently display the names and telephone numbers of all concerned family members, neighbors, and friends who will be available to help manage the inevitable critical periods. Include in the listings local police and fire departments, poison control hotlines, hospitals, and the physicians who attend the patient. Confirm that fire extinguishers and smoke detectors are fully operational.

Events that can cause dementia-like symptoms

As people age, there are many changes and losses that cause potent feelings of sadness and loneliness. These emotions are so powerful that they can disrupt thinking and impair memory. One of the most difficult life events is coping with the death of a spouse or other loved one.

CASE STUDY

Arthur, 69, had been a widower for several years when he lost his only son to cancer. They were partners in a small, fast-paced business and Arthur had hoped that just being at the plant all day would help to ease the pain that tormented him. That plan was unsuccessful.

He became profoundly sad, exhausted and these feelings bewildered and frightened him. Meanwhile, he was inattentive to his customers, neglected his stock, and delayed paying his bills. Withdrawn, confused and passive, Arthur began to let his business decline. Friends eventually avoided him because he rejected overtures of help and showed no interest in anything but speaking of his son's untimely death.

The hours and days immediately following a death of a loved one are filled with continuous, stressful activities. Then after the immediate pressures dissipate the bereaved person is overwhelmed with painful feelings of loneliness, or doubts about the medical care the loved one received, as well as the conflicting emotions of fear, guilt, and anger. The process of mourning is composed of all these thoughts and emotions. The mourning period is the external expression of these feelings and it is strongly influenced by the circumstances of the death, each individual's coping skills and spiritual beliefs, as well as the support of family and friends.

There is no time limit for grief, and the deeply personal way feelings are expressed is only one part of the intricate process of mourning. A positive step bereaved persons can take to regain control of their lives is to first reassess their health practices. For example, although the advice may sound almost trite, balanced nutrition is a dependable way to increase energy and some form of physical exercise, even just a daily walk, will help to reduce stress and may foster restful sleep at night. These two basic actions are the important first steps that can boost the immune system and improve overall health.

Grief that is intense and prolonged may be abnormal and should be professionally evaluated. After many months, Arthur's brother insisted they go together to seek medical advice and several therapeutic interventions were tried with some success. Eventually, Arthur also joined a recommended support group. These different strategies provided him with gradual relief from his depression. Relatives and friends of older people should be aware of the signs of depression among their older family members and friends, so they can assist them in obtaining treatment.

There are other major life changes besides a death in the family that can cause deeply felt emotional distress and adversely affect a person's mental or physical health. One of the more traditional is retirement. While most workers fantasize about extended leisure as being an extremely desirable aspect of retirement, there is much more to anticipate than limitless free time. After a few weeks of sleeping late and idling at home, most retirees find that they prefer some structure to their day and report that they like to keep busy.

Virtually all health care professional agree that social interaction and mental stimulation are essential aspects of retirement living. More important, as lifelong learning, mental and physical exercise, and staying engaged socially will nurture cognitive vitality, they are critical to optimal aging.

Once the restrictions of routine activities and obligations are lifted, many older adults flourish as never before because they now have the time and motivation to channel their energies, experiences and talents into rewarding, satisfying accomplishments.

Reversible and irreversible dementia

Most health care professionals know that an impaired memory is often an early symptom of dementia. However, forgetting someone's name or where a car is parked does not come under this heading. These incidents happen to everyone and although they may be frustrating, they are not signs of dementia.

Severe problems with thinking or memory are usually caused by any one of several diseases including Alzheimer's disease, Parkinson's, some vascular disorders and certain metabolic disorders. Other illnesses such as syphilis, acquired immune deficiency syndrome, multiple sclerosis and hypothyroidism may or may not lead to dementia, depending on the degree to which the brain is affected.

Although the majority of older adults show very little or no decline in their mental abilities, serious cognitive disorders such as Alzheimer's disease do increase in frequency as people age. Until medical science controls or eliminates those illnesses, as the oldest segment of the entire population of older adults keeps increasing, so will the demand for their specialized medical care.

The general term dementia is applied to individuals who are disabled because they have impaired intellectual abilities and related behavior disorders. There are at least 50 and possibly up to 100 causes of the disorder which can be either reversible or irreversible. Some causes of fully or partially **reversible** dementias are:

- drugs
- infections
- metabolic disorders
- nutritional deficiencies, particularly vitamin B12 and vitamin B1 (thiamine)
- vascular disorders
- brain tumor/brain injury
- depression
- chronic pain
- normal pressure hydrocephalus

drugs

Older adults are the leading consumers of medications. They account for about 30 percent of all prescriptions filled because they usually have several concurrent medical problems for which they take multiple medications. Elders taking any medications for pain, hypertension, depression, heart disease, or gastrointestinal disorders, need to be aware that <u>all</u> of these drugs can, under the right circumstances, produce the signs of dementia.

Alcoholism is another condition that causes dementia because alcohol slows brain activity and generates confusion and forgetfulness. The geriatric drinker may be a person who is increasing a bad habit the family always knew he had, or it could be someone's gentle grandmother who began to take just one drink to help get to sleep after her husband died and then later developed a drinking problem.

Alcohol is a drug and as such it can cause harmful effects when combined with prescriptions or over-the-counter medicine and, as the main consumers of medications, all elderly are at high risk for dangerous side effects.

infection

Any infection that attacks the brain can cause dementia. There are certain chronic illnesses, human immunodeficiency virus (HIV/AIDS) for example, that are known to frequently cause dementia. Nevertheless, if such illnesses as meningitis and encephalitis are effectively treated, that dreaded complication can often be prevented.

Recent nutritional research strongly suggests that nutritional supplements can also help to prevent infections. There is evidence indicating that daily vitamin/mineral supplements with additional zinc equal to a total dose of 20 mg./day, selenium to equal 100 micrograms, and 200 mg. of vitamin E daily can enhance immune function.

metabolic disorders

Virtually any disorder of the endocrine system, i.e., pituitary, adrenal, parathyroid, or thyroid glands, can trigger changes in the activity of the brain. One of the most common examples are those elderly individuals who have an underactive thyroid gland, a condition known as hypothyroidism, and display confusion as their primary symptom. A test of thyroid function is standard procedure when investigating some of the illnesses that cause dementia. Liver and kidney disorders can also affect the brain and produce dementia-type symptoms.

Other metabolic causes of dementia are anesthesia accidents and carbon monoxide poisoning. Dehydration of any older adult, with or without dementia, is the most common metabolic abnormality and it is also the easiest to correct.

nutritional deficiencies

It is well known that eating a balanced diet is essential for good health. Research has uncovered the link between a deficiency in the B complex vitamins, (thiamine, folate, niacin, and riboflavin) and a decrease in intellectual functioning.

There are also many drugs that can cause a decrease in appetite or a change in an older adult's taste perception. If these situations are unchecked they can give rise to inadequate nutrition.

Drugs that can cause loss of appetite	**Drugs that can cause changes in taste**
Chemotherapeutic drugs	Antidepressants
Amphetamines	Blood pressure medicines
Antibiotics	Antihistamines
Narcotics	Antipsychotics
Digitalis preparations	Muscle relaxants
Some cough and cold preparations	Alcohol

Table 1.3 classifications of drugs that alter appetite and taste.

Caregivers should consult with a physician and a pharmacist to learn if any of the drugs their family member is taking can have these side effects. It is also advisable to keep a monthly record of the individual's weight as a precaution.

A common barrier to good nutrition is poor dentition. Persons who have missing teeth or ill-fitting dentures cannot take advantage of many available wholesome foods. Poor nutrition and constipation often follow. Attention to oral hygiene and remedial dental care can further reduce causes of nutritional deficiencies.

Swallowing difficulties frequently develop as dementia advances. Nevertheless, nutritional needs can still be met by offering a soft diet consisting of ground or pureéd foods and thickened liquids and by crushing pills and mixing them with the food. All persons should learn the simple skill for choking rescue and any physician or nurse can instruct a caregiver to do this in a few minutes.

---

note

Confirm with the pharmacist if the action of a medication will be altered before crushing any pill or tablet.

---

vascular disorder

Ischemic damage to the brain, once termed arteriosclerosis, can cause a vascular dementia which, in the US and Europe, is the second most common cause of dementia following Alzheimer's disease.

---

note

In Japan vascular dementia accounts for 50 percent of all dementias that occur in individuals older than 65.

In Latin America 15 percent of all dementias are vascular and in Australia vascular and mixed dementia is 13 and 28 percent respectively.

A patient who has vascular dementia, commonly diagnosed as multi-infarct dementia (MID), characteristically has had a history of transient ischemic attacks (TIAs) with brief loss of consciousness, numbness or fleeting paralysis of an extremity, or transient blindness. If the TIA or mini-stroke occurs in an area of the brain responsible for memory and learning, then symptoms of memory loss and thinking problems become evident. This dementia usually follows cumulative damage to the brain due to hypertensive cardiovascular disease. Individuals with the disease may improve for short periods of time, then relapse. The prognosis for patients with MID is generally poor.

However, vascular dementia may be the most preventable form of dementia because the risk factors can be controlled with appropriate lifestyle changes. It is well known that hypertension can cause stroke which damages the brain. Older adults who control their hypertension can reduce the incidence of stroke or improve cognitive performance following stroke. Every older adult with hypertension is at risk for stroke.

Stroke - sometimes referred to as a "shock" or a "brain attack" - occurs when there is blockage of the circulation of blood to the brain. Stroke can also occur if a blood vessel in the brain ruptures spontaneously. Any interruption of the normal circulation of blood to the brain deprives that organ of oxygen and other vital nutrients, a development that can cause irreparable damage.

Stroke is an equal opportunity disease, affecting both men and women and its effects can be devastating. Men have slightly more strokes than do women, but most victims are women because women live longer. However, high blood pressure is a manageable disorder and the time and effort invested to gradually reduce blood pressure to appropriate levels can help to prevent a lifetime of disability.

Researchers have long believed that genes influence stroke risk and now, a recent study from the UK offers the best evidence that this is so. In the May, 2003 issue of Stroke, Paula Jerrard-Dunne, MRCPI, and colleagues from London's St. George's Hospital Medical School compared 1,000 stroke patients with 800 people who had no history of stroke or vascular disease. Compared with non-stroke patients, the stroke patients were more than twice as likely to have a parent or sibling who had suffered a stroke before age 66. Jerrard-Dunne and her team are currently refining the research to try and identify the specific genes associated with stroke.

Stroke is viewed as a risk factor for dementia since roughly one year after a stroke 25 percent of patients develop dementia for the first time.

brain tumor/brain injury

A brain tumor or abnormal growth can contribute to dementia if there is pressure on the blood vessels and nerves supplying the brain. Removal of a benign tumor will often cause the dementia to be reversed. Removal of malignant tumors is not as successful in reversing dementia. Trauma to the brain can also cause dementia depending on where the injury is located. These problems are diagnosed by using imaging techniques, e.g., CT scan or MRI..

depression

Depression (see chapter 2.) is the most common emotional illness affecting elderly persons and its symptoms are often confused with dementia. The Global Burden of Disease project determined that depression was the fourth leading cause of disability in 1990 worldwide, will be second only to heart disease in 2020. The project also revealed that undertreatment is widespread. The result is diminished functional capacity which further compromises the quality of life for affected older adults and their families. Depressed older adults have a greater risk of developing dementia. Furthermore, there is a direct association between depression and an increase in physical illnesses and disability, and ultimately an expanded use of health care resources.

chronic pain

Recent investigations of individuals with chronic pain and cognitive impairment uncovered compelling evidence confirming a link between the two symptoms. If an older adult is undermedicated for chronic pain there is a greater chance of dementia developing. Effective pain management not only enhances the patient's level of comfort but also may substantially reduce the incidence of cognitive impairment.

normal pressure hydrocephalus (NPH)

Normal pressure hydrocephalus occurs when there is an obstruction to the flow of cerebrospinal fluid. The blockage results in the compression of brain tissue and enlargement of the ventricles (spaces) in the brain. Some of the symptoms of NPH are incontinence, gait disturbance and dementia. NPH is treatable and is thought to account for five percent of all dementias

Some of the more prominent illnesses that cause **irreversible** dementia are:

- Alzheimer's disease
- Parkinsonism (paralysis agitans)
- Huntington's disease
- Lewy body dementia

Alzheimer's, Parkinson's, and Huntington's disease are all progressive and irreversible illnesses that share some common symptoms. Each illness, however, requires different treatment. Nevertheless, there is a common factor in the three diseases; virtually all the stricken patients experience high rates of depression.

Lewy body dementia is a disorder that occurs either alone or with Alzheimer's and Parkinsonism. This illness features hallucinations as well as wide fluctuations between confusion and lucidity. It gets its name from the abnormal protein deposits (the Lewy bodies) that are found in the brain after death upon autopsy.

Huntington's disease is hereditary and usually first appears in younger adults. The symptoms are characterized by a marked movement disorder and dementia. There are no effective treatments at this time.

Elders with any of these illnesses are usually aware of their gradual loss of intellectual abilities, a situation which is both frightening and frustrating.

Support for caregivers

Often overlooked are the caregivers who do not take adequate care of themselves because of the pressure and stress generated by their many responsibilities. Unsurprisingly, caregivers who are either spouses or adult children of elders also have higher-than-average rates of depression. In the United States, the National Family Caregiver Support Program (NFCSP) established in

November 2000 can help by providing:

- Individualized information on available resources to support caregivers.
- Assistance to families in finding services.
- Caregiver counseling, training, and peer support.
- Respite care.
- Limited supplemental

Information about the NFCSP in the U. S. may be obtained through a local Area Agency on Aging. The number is found in the telephone directory in the city or county government section under "Aging" or "Social Services".

International support information and services

A site that displays links for both practitioners and professionals is :www.aoa.gov Furthermore, for free access to an online caregivers' manual, click on to "National Family Caregiver Support Program", then "Caregiver Resources", then click on to "Because We Care".

Dementia Advocacy and Support Network. **http://www.dasninternational.org/index.html**

Caregiver Network, Inc., in Toronto is known internationally for providing information to families managing eldercare. **http://www.caregiver.on.ca/**

European Alzheimer Clearing House (EACH)

The European Alzheimer Clearing House aims to bring together initiatives in dementia care in the European Union in order to make better use of existing information and expertise. **http://www.each.be/**

Information about the NFCSP in the U. S. may be obtained through a local Area Agency on Aging. The number is found in the telephone directory in the city or county government section under "Aging" or "Social Services".

International support information and services

A site that displays links for both practitioners and professionals is :www.aoa.gov Furthermore, for free access to an online caregivers' manual, click on to "National Family Caregiver Support Program", then "Caregiver Resources", then click on to "Because We Care".

Dementia Advocacy and Support Network. **http://www.dasninternational.org/index.html**

Caregiver Network, Inc., in Toronto is known internationally for providing information to families managing eldercare. **http://www.caregiver.on.ca/**

European Alzheimer Clearing House (EACH) - The European Alzheimer Clearing House aims to bring together initiatives in dementia care in the European Union in order to make better use of existing information and expertise. **http://www.each.be/**

CHAPTER 2

Depression and the Older Adult

Depression is a mental disorder characterized by persistent sadness, decreased energy and loss of interest in activities. It is as much an illness as diabetes, cancer or heart disease. However, unlike those well recognized physical illnesses, depression in late life often is not diagnosed and treated promptly because the symptoms in older adults can easily be mistaken for dementia.

Depression can occur at any age but it is the most common of all mood disorders in the elderly. Although effective treatments exist, there are still barriers to identifying and treating depression, as well as other mental illnesses, in older adults. Consequently, when the disorder is left untreated, the cost in terms of pain, disability, and death is alarmingly high.

According to the World Health Organization (WHO), 121 million people worldwide suffer with depression Among adults over 60, it is among the eight most disabling medical conditions, <u>including</u> heart disease The effects of late life depression on older adults are even more severe in the following ways:

- It is the most reliable predictor of suicide in the elderly.
- It is a highly significant cause of disability and poor quality of life.
- When it coexists with physical disorders, the prognosis is poor.
- The illness increases the use of healthcare providers and facilities which results in escalating healthcare costs.

WHO also advises that depression is even more common than dementia. Its prevalence is found in the community to occur in as many as 15 - 25 percent of elders <u>particularly</u> if these older adults also have certain chronic illnesses as:

- heart disease
- stroke
- chronic pulmonary disease
- cancer
- Alzheimer's disease
- Parkinson's disease

note
More than 50 percent of residents in nursing homes and assisted living settings have late life depression.

Depression in the elderly has the potential to disrupt family life as well as imperil the life of the person who is ill; however, most of this suffering is unnecessary. The evidence is clear that treatment is effective almost 80 percent of the time. Why, then, are there so many elderly individuals with the disease undiagnosed and untreated? The reasons are many and varied:

- People with depression are reluctant to admit to a mental illness because of the perceived stigma. They may refuse help or delay timely treatment.
- Some families have the mistaken idea that it is normal for elderly individuals to feel depressed.
- The symptoms are often so disabling that the people affected cannot accurately describe their emotional pain and ask for help.
- Symptoms are easily misinterpreted by clinicians since they are usually described as physical complaints.
- Individual symptoms are treated, rather than the underlying cause.

Not only can depressive illness be found to coexist with several psychiatric disorders, certain medications can actually trigger its development. Moreover, there are other medical illnesses such as stroke, cancer, and chronic pulmonary diseases which are linked to the increased risk of depression developing. Depression can also appear at the same time as some of the sensory weaknesses normally seen old age, particularly the deficits of vision and hearing.

William is a 73 year old grandfather with hearing loss. Although he has hearing aids he seldom uses them; instead he relies most of the time on other ways of compensating for his deafness.

He thought he was handling his problem fairly well until the last time he went to his daughter's home to pick up his 4 year old grandson as he did each Thursday. As soon as he stepped into her house, his daughter told him that she was canceling the weekly trips to the park. "I'm sorry, Dad, I just don't think it's safe to let you to take Anthony. You might not hear him call if he needs you." William was stunned. Two years ago he lost his wife and the relationship with his grandson was a treasured source of comfort and joy. When he and the boy were together, he reveled in the boy's happiness and enjoyed a respite from his grief.

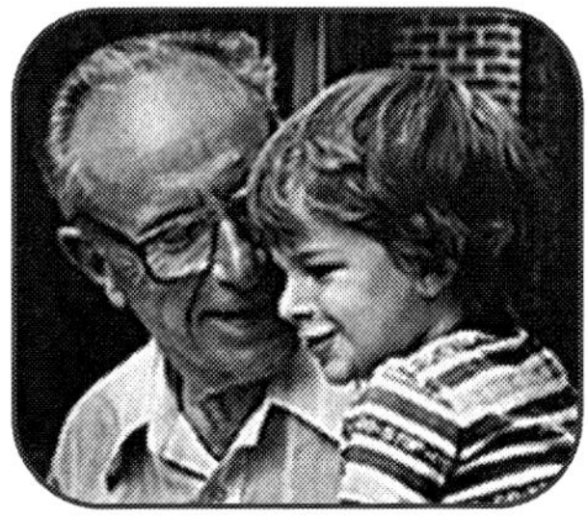

Source: NIH Word on Health, October 1999. www.nih.gov/news/WordonHealth/oct99/story02.htm

Since the special tie between him and his grandson was altered, William has been overcome with feelings of guilt and worthlessness. He has become withdrawn and dwells on the feeling that in some way, he deserves this "punishment". His family, although troubled by his apathy and occasional confusion, attribute the changes in his behavior to old age.

As mentioned in the previous chapter, depression refers to several disorders which are classified in the following ways:

- By their symptoms
- By the family's history
- By certain environmental factors, such as lack of education and poor working conditions
- By observing how the patient responds to treatment

Elderly individuals, like everybody else, experience periods of sadness commonly called the "blues", but these mood changes are usually temporary and benign. They are generally just normal reactions to some stress or worry which gets better with the support of family and friends. No further intervention is needed or even anticipated. However, clinical depression is much more serious and prolonged. When an older adult has this type of depression, families and health care workers need to understand that this is not a character flaw that could be changed if only the patient would make an effort. The stricken person is genuinely ill, and therefore it is pointless to make such statements as "pull yourself together" or "you can try harder". Such allegations can be compared to suggestions that cancer patients might try to control tumor growth with willpower.

Depression is a serious and sometimes dangerous medical condition to which older people as a group seem to be especially susceptible. Moreover, depressive illness can be difficult for clinicians to diagnose for several reasons:

- Some of the symptoms i.e. sleeplessness and poor appetite also occur in non-depressed older adults.
- Depressed moods are less noticeable in older adults.
- Physicians who are not psychiatrists may not be adequately trained to diagnose depressive illness.
- Depressed older adults usually visit their physicians with somatic complaints, e.g., they describe their problems in terms of bodily ailments. Toward that end, physicians assess a physical situation and prescribe treatment. However, this leaves the depression undiagnosed and consequently untreated.

Symptoms such as social withdrawal, confusion, reduction in energy, sleep disturbances, changes in appetite, and memory impairment apply to both dementia and depression. It takes an experienced, skilled clinician to distinguish between the two. However, dementia that is caused by depression is reversible. When the depression is treated, the confusion and memory impairment usually clears. Even if the physician determines that the patient has both depression and an irreversible dementia, the depression should be treated.

Families and friends need to be sensitive to the signs of depression in an older adult and take action when there are indications of persistent symptoms. Delaying or ignoring the evidence can result in exacerbated physical problems, disability, invalidism and ultimately, premature death.

Depression and the aging process

At one time depression was thought to be primarily a chemical imbalance caused by an inadequate supply of certain neurotransmitters, e.g., chemicals used to transmit messages throughout the cell network of the brain. The actual structure of the brain was assumed to be relatively unchanged by the process of aging. However, advanced imaging technology has plainly shown us that there are significant changes in the sizes of some of the brain sites where intellectual and emotional functions originate. In addition there are age-related alterations in the endocrine and immune systems that influence emotional response. These changes seem to explain why depression is found so often in the older adult.

Late life depression in some elders may also be a relapse of an early onset depression or the result of a strong genetic influence. Dominating the complex question of depression and the aging process should be the message that depression is a treatable medical illness and not a normal part of growing old.

Depression in the elderly can be hard to recognize because both patients and clinicians have lower functional expectations of senior citizens as a group. In our present social structure, we do not expect very much from persons who have retired.

Chapter 1. described the overlapping effects of various metabolic disturbances and the aging process on the brain. When depression exists in old age, the accompanying physical alterations and sensory losses an older adult endures often create psychosocial concerns and weighty medical problems that can contribute to depressive symptoms. Collectively, these issues also complicate treatment. Nonetheless, when properly diagnosed and treated most depressed elderly patients can improve and thereby enhance their quality of life enormously.

CAUSES OF DEPRESSION

A depressive illness is classed as either a primary or secondary disorder. A primary depression is one that is not caused by disease or a reaction to a drug. While this condition does exist in elderly individuals, it is not common.

Older adults are far more likely to experience a secondary depression, e.g., one that is caused either by a physical illness or as a side effect of medication. The latter is another reason why it is so important to accurately inform the primary physician of each drug, whether prescribed or over-the-counter, that the elderly individual is taking. The elderly are particularly vulnerable to the adverse effects of drugs because they experience more illnesses and, consequently, take more medications than any other age group. The slower metabolism of older adults and the large number of drugs they take virtually guarantees a drug reaction in some elders.

Vascular depression

Vascular depression is a disorder caused by changes in the blood flow in the brain. The symptoms of vascular depression are consistent with lesions in specific areas of the brain and physicians are able to confirm this through the interpretation of certain imaging tests. There is a link between depressed older adults and the occurrence of small strokes that do not produce the expected, physical symptoms generally associated with stroke, but do cause lesions on the brain. Dr. David Steffens of Duke University Medical Center who was involved in the research explains, "The type of depression these lesions are associated with is very different than depression in people in their 20s and 30s. The experience is much more of a losing of interest, apathy, and social withdrawal. The public and some physicians don't appreciate a criterion of slowing down compared to outward sadness or crying."

The investigators concluded that the patients had experienced "silent strokes", i.e. strokes that did not cause the customary symptoms of slurred speech or paralysis. However, the results also strongly suggested that whatever damage was done involved the parts of the brain controlling appetite, sleep, and energy. The changes produced typical depression symptoms: sleep disturbances, eating too much or too little, and apathy or fatigue.

The amount of depressive symptoms monitored in the research increased as the areas of damage to the brain increased. This was confirmed when the doctors conducted MRI's of the brain that allowed them to see finely detailed images.

Vascular depression is significant because it accounts for more than 40 percent of all depression in older adults. Moreover, it has the same risk factors as stroke which are:

- High blood pressure (hypertension)
- Obesity
- Lack of exercise
- Improper diet, which contributes to low HDL cholesterol and high LDL cholesterol
- Poorly managed diabetes
- Smoking

Most people know that stroke is a disease of the brain, but few understand the severity of the damage stroke can cause when it affects the entire body. There can be a wide range of severe disabilities such as paralysis, emotional problems, and impaired thinking and speaking.

The research findings about vascular depression are promising because each of the identified risks can be modified if the patient is willing to put in the time and effort. If lifestyle changes are improved in early adulthood, the chances of vascular depression developing are greatly reduced. Furthermore, these behavioral changes will also help to prevent stroke, the third leading cause of death in the United States.

DIFFICULTIES IN THE DIAGNOSIS AND TREATMENT OF GERIATRIC DEPRESSION

Geriatric depression, often referred to as late-life depression, differs from depression in the younger adult population. The depression that most older adults exhibit is influenced by the development of specific physical and psychological changes as is listed in table 2.1.

Change in:	**Symptom:**
Mood	Anxiety, agitation, despondency
Thought processes	Indecision, impaired memory, lack of concentration
Behavior	Social withdrawal; distrust, paranoia
Physical functioning	Alteration in sleep/wake pattern, i.e., sleeping too much or experiencing insomnia. Chronic fatigue. Decreased energy. Somatic complaints. Weight loss or gain.

Table 2.1 Changes in the depressed older adult.

Families become frustrated when they are unable to persuade an elderly relative to get help for these undesirable developments. They find that they have to make careful distinctions between supporting their loved one's independence and monitoring his health. If, for example, an elderly parent is not ready to accept advice, there are alternative approaches to try. Often a close friend, a sibling, or a clergyman can successfully intercede. If this approach fails, ask a physician to telephone the person directly. Many times a health professional will succeed by explaining the rewards of treating a health problem.

Some of the factors that confound the diagnosis of depression in older adults are:

- Families and clinicians may be misled by an elderly patient's description of vague, indistinct symptoms.
- Older adults focus more on bodily complaints rather than on their feelings.

- Symptoms of depression may be attributed to aging because less is expected of older adults after they retire.

- Both physician and patient concentrate on whatever chronic physical illness is present and the evaluation of depressive symptoms is easily overlooked.

- The stigma associated with depression, as with all mental illness, prevents many individuals from seeking treatment.

It frequently happens that the decision to seek treatment is left to a family member regardless of whether the situation is due to the slow progression of age or has reached a crisis. Families can support the depressed individual by remaining non-judgmental, answering questions honestly, validating the sadness and distress and using sincere listening skills. Although depression is a serious handicap at any age, it is harder to manage in old age for the following reasons:

- The health of the geriatric patient is usually poorer.

- The elderly have more medical problems that need treatment.

- Older adults lose family members and friends over the years and these losses weaken their support systems.

- Older adults risk a higher incidence of drug side effects.

- Depressive illness reduces the patient's incentive to comply with treatment.

- Elderly individuals generally do not respond well to antidepressant therapy.

A physician will have suggestions and information appropriate in these situations. Also, The National Institute of Mental Health has free publications and fact sheets available online at:

www.nimh.nih.gov/ or

NIMH Public Inquiries
6001 Executive Boulevard, Rm. 8184, MSC 9663
Bethesda, MD 20892-9663 U.S.A.
Voice: (301) 443-4513, Fax: (301) 443-4279
TTY: (301) 443-8431

International resources are available at :
http://www.alzheimers.org.uk/

or by writing to:

Alzheimer's Society, Gordon House, 10 Greencoat Place, London, SW1P 1PH
Tel: 020 7306 0606 (Intl +44 (0) 20 7306 0606)
Fax: 020 7306 0808
Email: **enquiries@alzheimers.org.uk**

http://www.alz.co.uk/help/associations.html is a site that lists all countries alphabetically with name, address, telephone and fax numbers, email addresses and websites.

In spite of the fact that depressive symptoms in older people are often missed, most health professionals are learning to better identify and treat the depressive illness. They know that some symptoms may be side effects of medication the older person is taking for a physical problem, or that they can be caused by a coexisting illness. If a diagnosis of depression is made, treatment with medication and/or psychotherapy will help the depressed person return to a happier, more fulfilling life.

The difference between depression and grief

It is all too common for older adults to lose family members and friends over the years. However, there is a substantial difference between the sadness due to mourning and the despair of depression.

Everyone readily equates depression with sadness and grief implies sadness. It is an expected and normal reaction after the death of a loved one. Those who are grieving usually are consoled and supported by family and friends, as well as by being comforted by their religious beliefs and the passage of time. However, the pain of the clinically depressed can only be relieved by medical treatment.

Clinical depression is an illness that affects an individual's body, mood, and reasoning. It influences thought processes and self esteem as well as appetite and sleep habits. Depressive disorders are not signs of personal shortcomings nor are they benign emotional disturbances. The characteristic physical symptoms of depression are vague aches and pains which are hard to describe and do not respond satisfactorily to treatment. The following behaviors are typical warning signs of depression:

- Prolonged despondency, anxious, or "empty" mood.
- Feelings of hopelessness.
- Feelings of guilt, worthlessness, helplessness.
- Loss of interest or pleasure in pastimes and activities that were once enjoyed.
- Lack of energy, increased fatigue.
- Decreased ability to concentrate, remember, follow directions, or make decisions.
- Insomnia or sleeping too much.
- Marked changes in appetite which lead to weight loss or gain.
- Thoughts of death or suicide; suicide attempts.
- Persistent restlessness, irritability.

If any of these signs are identified in an elderly person, it is time for a medical evaluation. (Please see appendix 2. For a sample geriatric depression scale)

THE DEPRESSED ELDER IN LONG TERM CARE

By some estimates, more than 25 percent of nursing home residents and more than 15 percent of elders hospitalized with hip fractures or heart disease have or will develop, depression.

Family members who visit depressed elderly relatives in hospitals or nursing homes can still be very helpful to their loved one in the following ways:

1. Understand that the patient is not responsible for his feelings. Do not try to coax him out of any negative feelings.

2. Offer the nursing home resident choices in order to allow some measure of control. For example, say "do you want to see today's movie or shall we just sit and talk?" Or "do you need a sweater or are you warm enough?"

3. Be a good listener. When you are focused on the resident and his conversation, it reinforces the message that he is important.

4. Allow for spiritual expression. Prayer can be a comfort and a source of inner peace. Even if religion has not been important in the past, do not assume that is still the situation. Introduce the subject non-judgmentally as a topic of casual conversation and listen to the response.

5. If you hear the resident say, "I might as well be dead!" Validate, do not dismiss the statement by saying, "oh, you really don't mean that." At that moment, he really does mean that. Instead, try saying "you must really feel very unhappy (or very uncomfortable) to say that. Help me to understand what is troubling you."

Lisa visited her chronically ill and depressed mother-in-law several times a week to help her with her meals. Although the elderly lady had been living in a nursing home for 3 years, she never accepted the fact that she was unable to care for herself in her own home.

As soon as Lisa had her coat off, her mother-in-law would greet her with the same mournful exclamation: "Well, I guess the next step is the cemetery!" But instead of looking dismayed and denying that the old lady in the wheelchair really meant what she said, Lisa would give her a hug, smooth the coverlet over her knees, and say, "Mom, you don't sound good to me. Do you need something for pain? Are you warm enough?" And eventually she would hear her mother-in-law sigh heavily and say something like, "oh, I guess I'll make it through another day." At that point, Lisa would get the tray and prepare to feed her.

By acknowledging what the older woman said, inquiring about her comfort and touching her in a caring manner, Lisa communicated both verbally and non-verbally her genuine concern for her mother-in-law's well being.

The move into a nursing home causes major emotional difficulties for both the residents and their families. The residents feel some sadness and anxiety and most of the families bear a burden of guilt. It can be helpful to remind the resident of the many hardships they endured in the past, and ask them how they coped. This approach provides an opportunity to reinforce the fact that although the circumstances are different now, the same inner strength and coping skills that helped years ago is still within them.

Families can benefit by networking with others in similar situations through support groups to learn strategies for managing their frustrations and understanding their guilt.

BEREAVEMENT AND DEPRESSION

Although the symptoms of depression and the grief during the bereavement period have many similarities, the two are separate and distinct emotions. The loss of a spouse, for example, generates intensely stressful feelings. The debilitating sadness experienced by the surviving partner is a painful, but admittedly natural, reaction to death. Those who have lost loved ones readily acknowledge that the signs of grief include most of the following:

- Crying
- Insomnia/excessive sleeping
- Loss of appetite/overeating
- Confusion
- General anxiety
- Apathy
- Social withdrawal

Many professionals believe that the grief caused by the death of a loved one can heighten an individual's physical or emotional disorders. Charlton and colleagues at the Centre for Primary Health Care Studies in Warwick, UK suggest that bereavement can be viewed as a medical problem since their research showed that prescriptions increased for both physical and emotional illness following death of a family member. However, they caution clinicians not to over-medicalize grief.

Although the symptoms of grief are the same as those of depression, the major difference is that in grief they fluctuate for a period of time, then gradually abate. Conversely, there is no relief from the despondency of untreated depressive illness.

When Lorraine lost her husband, she was inconsolable. Most of the time she was in bed sleeping, yet she was always tired. She endured crying spells, lack of appetite, and had difficulty concentrating. A few months later, Lorraine realized with some surprise that there were some days she felt almost normal; and then all of a sudden, like a huge ocean wave, grief would wash over her and she would revert to a state of despair. As the months went by, however, Lorraine noted that the really bad times weren't happening as often.

If sadness persists unabated for two months or more the bereaved individual may have a depressive illness. During the first year of being widowed, more than 20 percent of the surviving spouses will actually develop a clinical depression. Left untreated, this disorder often progresses to a chronic state because it disrupts both endocrine and immune function. The result is that the general health of the depressed older adult is unnecessarily damaged. Although bereavement itself is not labeled a mental disorder, if the abnormal symptoms are prolonged then the health of the affected individual can be seriously impaired. Bereavement symptoms that are not addressed can be debilitating and they place elderly people at risk for depression, which in turn, is linked to death from heart attack, suicide or other causes.

Early intervention can deflect a potentially life-threatening disorder. There is much that can be done through formal treatment, support group participation, or a combination of the two to ease the symptoms of depression that arises from bereavement.

RISKS OF UNRECOGNIZED, UNTREATED DEPRESSION

Untreated depression becomes a chronic disability and causes needless suffering for individuals and their families. More important, untreated depression can be fatal. Findings cited in the medical literature clearly indicate that elderly persons with depressive symptoms are more prone to cardiac fatalities than a similar population of individuals who are not depressed. The American Journal of Cardiology reports that mild depression after an acute heart attack raises the mortality risk 5 times that of the non-depressed individual. Moderately depressed patients have nearly 10 times the risk!

Furthermore, depression has also been found to coexist with a large number of patients who have diabetes or osteoporosis, two disorders that are widespread among mature adults.

---

note

Scientists have known for several years that the bone mineral density of women with a history of major depression is 10 to 15 percent lower than normal for their age.

The possibility of suicide by depressed older adults is another critical concern. Although most of the people who commit suicide are depressed, the link between suicide attempts and depression is complex. It is safe to say, however, that a truly hopeless individual is more at risk for this type of destructive behavior than someone who looks forward to the future.

The National Institute of Mental Health warns that there is undisputed evidence showing major depression to be a significant predictor of suicide and older adults to be the group most at risk.

Americans 65 and older account for approximately 20 percent of all suicides. What is not widely known, though, is that in the US the highest incidence of suicide is found in elderly white males aged 85 and older. Szanto, Gildengers et al report in Drugs and Aging 2002 that in almost all industrialized countries, men 75 years and older have the highest suicide rate among all age groups.

---

note

About 30,000 deaths annually are authentic suicides. The actual number is probably much higher since many deaths caused by suicide are officially ruled accidental.

Many geriatric suicide victims were seen by their primary care physicians a short time before the fatality. The results of a suicide treatment survey suggested that one reason for deferring the treatment of melancholy, despondent elders might be an age bias on the part of some clinicians who saw the depressed older adults. This was surely not intentional, rather, it reflected the lack of geriatric training available in today's medical schools.

The physicians surveyed acknowledged that their geriatric patients talked about hopelessness and death, but they were reluctant to use medication or to suggest psychotherapy because they considered the symptoms of guilt and worthlessness that they observed to be normal for aged individuals. In addition, many of the physicians were unsure of their diagnostic skills. Furthermore, few were confident about prescribing antidepressants and most replied that they didn't feel that therapy would be helpful.

Other clinicians pointed out that the time constraints imposed by managed care regulations sharply restricted the duration of the office visit necessary to complete meticulously detailed medical and social histories so essential for an accurate diagnosis.

The policy of most primary care physicians, (PCPs) however, is far more positive. Recent studies show that increasing numbers of PCPs have been prescribing antidepressants for their elderly patients A combination of factors is probably responsible for this shift, e.g.:

- A new class of of antidepressants – the selective serotonin reuptake inhibitors – (SSRIs) which have fewer side effects than earlier antidepressants.
- Increased recognition of depression by PCPs .
- Financial incentives leading to increased reliance on antidepressants instead of more costly psychotherapy.

emotional symptoms:	physical symptoms:
anxiety	sleeping more or less than usual
feelings of guilt	eating more or less than usual
restlessness, irritability	excessive fatigue
marked lack of interest in formerly pleasurable experiences	recurring headaches, stomach aches
feelings of worthlessness, of being unloved	chronic pain
feelings of despair	lethargy, indifference

Table 2.2 significant symptoms of depression.

In order to ensure treatment for a depressed older adult, families must be proactive. An adult child of a depressed elder, for example, may have to vigorously assume the role of advocate and insist on more aggressive care for the depressed elderly parent whose mental health needs are not being fully met.

In order to encourage questions about behavior and mood and productive discussions between patients and clinicians, the National Institute of Mental Health (NIMH) online at **www.nimh.nih.gov/** recommends that the following symptoms be investigated by a health care professional:

The National Institute of Mental Health can also be reached at:

NIMH Public Inquiries
6001 Executive Boulevard, Rm. 8184, MSC 9663
Bethesda, MD 20892-9663 U.S.A.
Voice (301) 443-4513; Fax (301) 443-4279
TTY (301) 443-8431

The Karolinska Institutet maintains an electronic library of international links to resources and practice guides for laypersons and professionals at: **http://www.mic.ki.se/Diseases/f3.html**

Inquiries may also be made at:

Karolinska Institutet, Library, P.O.Box 200 S-171 77 Stockholm, Sweden
Tel: +46-8-728 80 00, Fax: +46-8-34 87 06, E-mail: info@kib.ki.se

In the past, few people suspected that the causes for the increased sickness and death of older adults with depression could have a physical basis. However, clinical investigators who have been examining the circumstances of death in this population have discovered the following biologic factors to be contributory:

- There is an increase in the production of stress hormones
- Heart rhythms are found to be irregular
- There is an increase in the viscosity (stickiness) of the blood which causes clots to develop.
- The immune system is weaker.

These features are additional reminders that unrecognized, untreated depression can cause system-wide bodily malfunctions and a cascade of threatening health problems.

---

note
By some estimates, nearly 50 percent of older adults experience late life depression for a period of time.

RISK FACTORS FOR DEPRESSION

The person who is aware of the risk factors for depression can be one step ahead of a mental health problem. Generally, the risks are placed in four categories:

1. genetic
2. biochemical
3. environmental
4. social/psychological issues

genetic factors

Depression may run in families, and children of depressed parents are more likely at higher risk for developing the disease.

biochemical factors

When an individual experiences a depressive illness the chemistry of the brain is disrupted. Specifically, there is a drop in levels of neurotransmitters, those important chemicals that nerve networks rely on for the transmission of information within the brain. Lesions have also been seen in the area of the brain governing emotions.

environmental and other stressors

The death of a loved one, a move to a new neighborhood, or a retirement can trigger depression. Moreover, certain illnesses such as Parkinson's disease, stroke or cancer and the development of any physical impairments, ex. incontinence or vision and hearing deficits, also have strong links to depression. It is well known that there is a relationship between substance abuse and individuals who have depression. In the case of older adults, the substance abused is usually alcohol. Polypharmacy, which is widespread among the elderly, can also cause depressive symptoms.

social/psychological traits

Certain personality characteristics namely poor self esteem, a tendency toward worrying excessively, and holding a persistently negative viewpoint describe individuals who are more susceptible to depression. These are traits found in people who haven't developed the ability to prioritize their problems or to cope with the many challenges of daily living.

There are some basic, common-sense, steps people can take to lower the risks of developing depression:

1. Prepare for the major changes in life such as retirement or the deaths of family or friends. Develop and maintain friendships over the years. Friends help provide comfort and support when people are bereaved. The cultivation of other interests and pastimes which keep the mind and body active and thereby limit any effects of depression is an extremely important practice.

2. Maintain physical fitness and eating a balanced diet, two fundamental habits to develop in order to in avoid illnesses that can cause disability or depression.

3. Follow directions to the letter if taking any medication because depression is a side effect that is associated with many drugs. Question a pharmacist when there are anydoubts about a prescription.

The non-professional's insight into depression

How can a layman reliably distinguish between the normal sadness that follows the loss of a loved one and the feelings of hopelessness that are caused by certain physical limitations? The simplest method is for families to monitor the elderly relative for the following common warning signs of depression:

- Chronic fatigue
- Marked change in appetite
- Change in sleep habits
- Frequent crying
- Irritability and anxiety
- Lack of interest in everyday activities
- Guilt feelings
- Thoughts of death

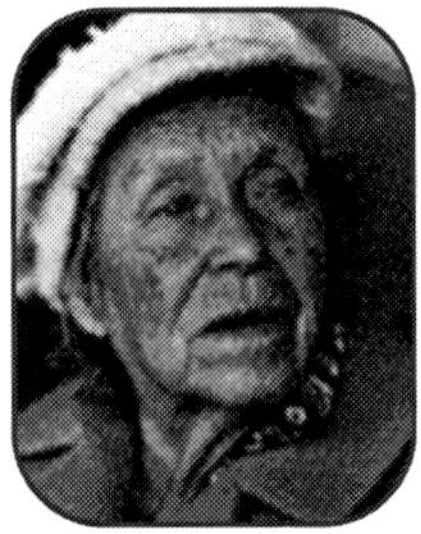

Figure 2.1
Source: Images of Aging, Administration on Aging, National Aging Information Center

Depressed older adults have also been known to leave obvious clues for family, friends or health professionals. For example, careless hygiene, indifference to family functions and activities, and change in appetite are all possible signs of depression. More important, these are often warnings that the situation is abnormal and the elderly individual needs professional help.

Estelle, 82, a retired bookkeeper, had long been used to making her own decisions. The thought of being dependent on anyone, either physically or emotionally, was abhorrent to her.

However, in the past two years she has been involved in several minor traffic accidents. Her problems began to escalate when she backed into a car across the street as she exited her driveway and caused considerable and costly damage to her neighbor's vehicle. A month later on a rainy morning she ran over her own mailbox at the end of her driveway. Since then she sustained a series of dents and scrapes in parking lots.

However, the unthinkable happened two months ago. Estelle stopped to pick up her friend on the way to church as was her custom each Sunday morning. When she thought her friend was in the car, she began to slowly pull away. Unfortunately, the woman still had one foot on the pavement. Her friend was knocked to the ground and suffered a fractured hip. Estelle's horrified sons reacted swiftly by confiscating both her keys and her car.

But the unthinkable happened to her friend has caused Estelle profound sorrow and regret. Adding to her acute sense of guilt and humiliation is the distress she feels about her sons' abrupt decision that she is no longer a competent driver. She has lost weight and has become withdrawn and lethargic. She seldom goes out of her house and often does not answer the phone.

ILLNESSES ASSOCIATED WITH DEPRESSION

As mentioned earlier, depressive illness is often unrecognized and untreated when it coexists with another disorder. Nonetheless, it is a distinct illness and requires specific treatment.

Any discussion of depression would be incomplete if the following chronic illnesses were not mentioned, as they are often associated with depression:

- Parkinson's disease (PD)
- Alzheimer's disease (AD)
- Stroke
- Diabetes
- Cancer
- Thyroid disorders
- Cushing's disease

These treatable medical conditions are most frequently linked with the onset of depression.

---

note

Depression can precede the symptoms of Parkinson's.

There is a strong positive association between depression and the subsequent incidence of Parkinson's disease.

Treatment of coexisting depression can have a positive effect on the course of the medical illness, especially when it improves a person's ability to comply with the management of certain chronic illnesses such as diabetes and heart disease. Furthermore, it can significantly enhance an individual's quality of life and that of the family.

The prompt treatment of depression yields the best results, whereas the typical consequences of delayed treatment are a poor response and a resistance to improvement. Overlooking or misidentifying depressive illness in elderly persons frequently results in nursing home placement because these individuals become so disabled that families feel helpless to improve the situation. They come to the reluctant decision that caring at home for their impaired relative is no longer possible, and that only long term care can meet the patient's needs. At that point, the older adult is labeled as suffering from dementia and may not receive appropriate treatment for depressive illness.

CHAPTER 3

Alzheimer's Disease

Alzheimer's disease (AD) has been called both "the long goodbye" and a "silent epidemic". It is a "long goodbye" because during the slow, protracted course of the disease as the subtle initial symptoms are ebbing and flowing, there are just occasional hints of the course of this terminal illness. As the disease advances, personality is altered and disability increases to the extent that the very essence of the individual is fundamentally changed. Eventually, the patient is almost unrecognizable to his family. It is a "silent epidemic" because the World Health Organization (WHO) estimates that 37 million people worldwide have dementia and more than half have AD. In a fact sheet issued in December, 2001, WHO stated that about 5 percent of men and 6 percent of women over 60 years of age are affected with Alzheimer's. This figure is projected to increase rapidly over the next 20 years as the number of people with AD doubles every five years after age 65. In the US, one in 10 people over 65 and nearly half of those over 85 suffer from Alzheimer's disease. Currently, at least 4 million Americans have the condition. That number could jump to 14 million by the year 2050 unless preventive measures are developed.

Edward Truschke, president of the Alzheimer's Association National Office in the US, declared that "we have an imminent worldwide epidemic", when referring to the growing aging population and the prevalence of the disease.

Although AD is the most common cause of dementia among people age 65 and older, the disease can occur in people in their 40's and 50's. Individuals with early onset AD have the same symptoms as older adults with the illness. The main difference is the way the disease affects the life of a middle-aged adult (under 50) since someone in this age range may still have parental responsibilities. Consequently, both spouse and children need to understand the changes they see in the patient and learn how to function together as a family during this time of physical and emotional upheaval. In addition, the patient with early onset AD is probably still employed. As a result the problems caused by the inevitable cognitive decline usually damage workplace relationships and performance. The younger AD patient may be viewed as lazy, disinterested, undependable or unstable. He could be terminated for emotional or psychiatric reasons instead of acquiring a diagnosis that could qualify as a medical disability. The subsequent loss of income causes a devastating crack in the family's economic base.

Symptoms

The subtle age-related and irreversible brain disorder called Alzheimer's causes memory loss, behavioral and personality changes, and a decline in the ability to think, plan and reason. The preliminary signs of forgetting and minor personality alterations are barely noticeable because the symptoms unfold so slowly. Initially, the person affected has some trouble remembering, peoples' names, the names of familiar objects and recent events. However, since there is no marked change in physical appearance these atypical developments are readily excused by families and friends as caused by stress, or even a normal reaction to growing older. Families may dismiss erratic behavior and other abnormal signs out of fear or ignorance. This position is frustrating to all in the health care community because although the cause and cure of AD are still unknown, there is promising treatment available that can often improve the patient's quality of life and ease family stress.

Memory loss that impairs one's everyday activities is never a part of normal aging. Rather, it is symptomatic of dementia, a condition which also includes disorganized intellectual functioning, diminished language skills and poor judgment. The alteration and loss of brain cells distinguishes AD from other causes of dementia and is the hallmark of this disease, the most common of all dementing illnesses.

As part of their mission to provide information, care and support as early as possible to people with AD and their families, the Alzheimer's Association lists ten warning signs for family caregivers and friends:

1. **Memory loss.** Newly acquired information is forgotten more often than usual. Memory loss is also displayed by asking the same questions repeatedly.
2. **Difficulty performing familiar tasks.** As an example, an AD patient may no longer remember how to shave himself or start his car.
3. **Problems with language.** Common, everyday words are forgotten.
4. **Disorientation to time and place.** AD patients forget where they are and how they got there.
5. **Poor judgment.** Those with Alzheimer's may dress inappropriately i.e., wearing insufficient clothing on a cold day.
6. **Problems with abstract thinking.** Balancing a checkbook or handling any financial transaction becomes unmanageable. Numbers are virtually meaningless.
7. **Misplacing things.** A person with Alzheimer's disease may put things in unsuitable places, such as placing a sandwich under a pillow.
8. **Changes in mood and behavior.** Rapid mood swings are also characteristic of AD patients. An individual with AD can be calm, then suddenly break into tears or become angry for no apparent reason.

9. **Changes in personality.** Although the personalities of elders may change slightly with age, persons with Alzheimer's undergo marked alterations. They often become very confused, paranoid, fearful and dependent.

10. **Loss of initiative.** It is normal for anyone to tire of their obligations from time to time. The AD patient, however, becomes indifferent to responsibilities and relationships. He appears to be passive, apathetic and withdrawn.

A person with two or three of these warning signs requires medical help. Early diagnosis is an invaluable first step in securing appropriate treatment, care and support services. Families also need to be aware that medications as well as secondary illnesses such as strokes or depression often mimic the dementia of AD. The advantage of early detection is that it allows time for families to study treatment options and plan ahead financially and legally. Being able to make these decisions empowers the patient at a time when he is vulnerable and feels completely defenseless.

Alzheimer's is one of a group of disorders referred to as 'dementias', and although the risk of developing AD increases with age, neither AD nor any dementia can be considered normal for elderly individuals. All dementing illnesses, including AD, are caused by disorders that affect the brain. When there is no disease, the human brain is perfectly capable of functioning well into the tenth decade of life.

Seventy eight year old Nancy decided to visit her daughter who lived about 3 miles away. She got into her car and drove directly to her daughter's home. When she pulled into the driveway she sat quietly for several minutes staring blankly at the house. Then she abruptly backed out of the driveway. Several hours later a state trooper found her parked on the side of a busy highway. She did not know how to turn off the ignition. Nancy could not explain to the officer what she was doing there, nor could she tell him where she lived.

A few years ago there was a story in the news about an elderly couple found in a small Canadian town asleep and huddled together in a car. The incident happened in late December, on a bitter cold evening. Apparently they had driven all the way from Maine but neither of them knew how or why they ended up in Canada. They had simply run out of food, money, and finally, gas.

These true cases are typical examples of the cognitive decline characteristic of Alzheimer's, a disease originally described by a German physician named Alois Alzheimer in 1906. His journals contained notes documenting the world's first known case of the disease and the patient portrayed in these notes exhibited many of the symptoms still seen today. When he examined the patient's brain after her death, Alzheimer found abnormal deposits of protein (amyloid plaques) and nerve cells that appeared as tangled bundles of fibers (neurofibrillary tangles). These plaques and tangles have become AD's classic benchmarks. It is now known that this damage develops first in the areas of the brain used for memory and other cognitive functions.

The journals also poignantly document the fact that the patient was acutely aware of experiencing her eroding intellect and terrifying personality changes. One keenly sensitive entry is the patient's quote, "I have lost myself" , and clearly, Alzheimer's is all about loss.

CAUSES

The causes of Alzheimer's disease are not fully understood but the combination of expanded brain research and the increased scientific investigation of AD has uncovered links between certain genes and Alzheimer's. As an example, a genetic defect seems to be inherited in a some families where early onset AD (before age 50) has been documented for several generations. However, only 5 percent of Alzheimer's disease is early onset.

There are many theories, but no single definitive cause has been discovered in the cases of the other 95 percent of AD victims who exhibit the symptoms after age 65. The prevailing explanation is that a combination of genetic and environmental factors trigger the disease. Potential causes under investigation are:

neurotransmitter deficiency Neurotransmitters are chemicals in the brain that enable nerves in different parts of the brain to send messages to each other. Acetylcholine is a neurotransmitter that plays a pivotal role in memory formation and, in the case of AD, there is a dramatic decrease in its supply.

environmental factors Environmental factors being investigated range from the use of anesthetics and other drugs to food-borne toxins.

genetic factors or predispositions As mentioned earlier, a clear genetic link has been identified in the small number of early-onset AD cases. Two other genetic theories investigated by researchers have recently yielded compelling evidence of their link to AD: one is the influence of *apolipoprotein E* and the other is the effect of elevated *homocysteine* levels.

The more common form of Alzheimer's occurs late in life and as yet no clear family tie has been proven. A risk factor for this type of AD is a protein called apolipoprotein E (apoE), a substance that helps to transport cholesterol in the blood. There are, however, three versions of the protein; apoE2, apoE3 and apoE4. Of the three, research indicates that persons with apoE4 are most likely to develop AD.

A recent issue of the New England Journal of Medicine announced some promising new AD research results. The findings in the report pointed to a strong association between high plasma homocysteine levels and significant memory loss. Homocysteine is an amino acid long known to be linked to coronary artery disease, stroke, and venous blood clots. The results of the landmark study clearly showed that people with elevated levels of homocysteine in the blood had nearly double the risk of developing Alzheimer's disease. Other theories about the causes of Alzheimer's suggest either an unidentified virus or a lack of nerve growth factor, a substance that promotes the development of new nerve connections. Researchers also are investigating the role of the hormone estrogen in AD as well as the effects of inflammation on brain activity. The latter explains the recent interest in nonsteroidal anti-inflammatory drugs (NSAIDs) and their role in slowing the progression of the disease.

Research has shown that a number of inflammatory processes are active in the brains of patients with AD. These findings lead scientists to believe that an anti-inflammatory regimen may offer some neuroprotection. Dr. Paul Aisen, Director of Memory Disorders at Georgetown University, claims in the Journal of Pain Symptom Management, claims that there is evidence suggesting that inflammation in the brain may contribute to AD damage. Examples of NSAIDs being studied that might help slow the progression of Alzheimer's are rofecoxib and naproxen.

Most discussions about Alzheimer's disease includes questions about aluminum and it's effect on the brain. It is known that aluminum is toxic, but does it contribute to Alzheimer's disease? The aluminum toxicity theory was popular in the mid-sixties after researchers injected aluminum salts into animals that subsequently caused changes in the animal brains that were similar to the changes observed in the brains of AD patients. While the changes were not identical, discussion of the similarity was misinterpreted by the public. Widespread fears caused people to discard their aluminum cookware and avoid products made with baking powder as well as certain antacids and deodorants known to contain aluminum. In the 1980's painstaking research studies by Markesbery and Ehmann revealed no relationship between AD and the amount of aluminum found in human brains.

PROTECTION

As public information about the incidence of AD increased, questions have been raised by informed adults about measures to take to avoid developing the disease. It is well known, for example, that many risk factors for stroke can be altered by lowering blood pressure, stopping smoking and exercising regularly. Although existing hypertension can be controlled by medication, for most individuals the adoption of a healthier lifestyle would probably be enough to prevent the onset of hypertension. This would include adhering to a nutritious diet and exercise plan, maintaining near ideal body weight, avoiding tobacco and excessive alcohol, and controlling stress.

The general public can readily learn how to achieve a healthy lifestyle since virtually all media frequently imparts information about what constitutes good health. But what precautions can an individual take to ensure reasonably healthy <u>intellectual</u> functioning in old age? At the present time there is no pill or diet that science has to offer to successfully prevent the development of Alzheimer's disease. However, there does seem to be a strong association between an individual's level of education and the risk of developing AD. Several studies have revealed that the more education a person has, the less chance there is of Alzheimer's disease developing. David Snowdon, author of Aging With Grace, writes that "most of the large studies throughout the world have found links between lower levels of education and Alzheimer's". Margaret Gatz, professor of psychology at the University of Southern California proposes that the greater levels of educational achievement may act as a cushion against intellectual impairment.

One obvious benefit education can offer is learning how to live a healthier lifestyle. There is a link, for example, between the incidence of AD and the amount of fat a person eats. Therefore, it would be prudent to restrict the intake of animal fat in the diet. A diet that consists of a healthy balance of nutrients and includes low levels of saturated fat and cholesterol is associated with a lower risk of mental impairment. To a large degree, good mental health depends on good physical health. Exercise is also known to improve the circulation in the brain because the increased blood flow delivers essential nutrients that keep brain tissue healthy.

note

Ginkgo is a popular supplement widely advertised as being effective for enhancing memory. The August 21, 2002 JAMA issue has discredited this claim. Yet the herb continues to generate controversy. More recently the British Alzheimer's Society announced that a major review of clinical trials provides promising evidence that the dietary supplement Gingko biloba can improve memory and function in people with dementia.

The folic acid link

People who have Alzheimer's disease often have low levels of folic acid (folate) in their blood, but it is not clear whether this is a result of the disease or if they are simply malnourished because of their illness. Scientists theorize that consuming adequate amounts of folic acid - in the diet or by supplementation - could be beneficial to the aging brain and help protect it against AD and other neurodegenerative diseases.

Folic acid has also been found to reduce elevated homocysteine levels in most people. Since there is a relationship between high homocysteine levels and Alzheimer's, there should be an effort to reduce these levels by increasing intake of folate and vitamins B6 and B12.

Green leafy vegetables, citrus fruits and juices, whole wheat bread and dried beans are good sources of the vitamins. Since 1998 the Food and Drug Administration in the U. S. has required the addition of folic acid to enriched breads, cereals, flours, corn meals, pastas, rice and other grain products. However, because the symptoms of AD take a long time to manifest themselves, researchers speculate that it will be many years before folate supplementation in food could have a demonstrable effect on the incidence of dementia.

The influence of mental activity

Older adults are also encouraged to keep mentally active by participating in pastimes that test their memories, problem-solving skills and judgment. As examples, working crossword puzzles, playing cards and board games, are all good cognitive exercises. Learning a new skill, such as how to use a computer, or play a musical instrument are other intellectual challenges that elders can find personally rewarding and intellectually stimulating. Many researchers firmly believe that cognitive activity can help to reduce a person's chance of developing Alzheimer's. There are recent clinical findings that support this view as seen in the February, 2002 issue of Journal of the American Medical Association. Scientists strongly suggest that people who are more intellectually active may develop connections among neurons that reduce the risk of the brain being affected by the disease.

---

note

Testosterone may play a role in the mental acuity in men as they age. Older men with high testosterone levels seem to have better memory and concentration skills. It is unclear how testosterone acts on the brain and more research needs to be done on this hormone.

DIAGNOSIS

Expanded neurological research has revealed many of the complex activities of the brain and related how they influence behavior. Previously the examination of brain tissue at autopsy was the definitive test to confirm the diagnosis of AD. However, a newly developed test combines the use of a PET scan (positron emission tomography) and the injection of a chemical tracer to identify brain lesions associated with AD. Although this research is extremely promising, the average cost of a PET scan is about $1500 and as yet the cost is seldom covered by insurance. Nevertheless, physicians still reach a highly probable diagnosis in about 90 percent of the AD patients who display symptoms of the disease. They do this by taking a complete health history, doing a comprehensive physical exam, conducting neurological and mental status assessments as well as other related laboratory tests and imaging studies.

Some of the following questions are examples of information needed for a health history:

- How and when did the problems begin?
- Have the symptoms worsened?
- Do they vary from day to day?
- How long have they lasted.?

A mental status examination (MSE) is another key component of diagnostic process. However, any MSE must be used with caution since certain factors need to be weighed before drawing firm conclusions: e.g., patient's level of education or primary language. etc. (For more information about mental status exams, please see Chap. 1, p.14.)

It is advisable to have a family member or trusted friend along to confirm or supplement information given. The physical examination is a critical component of the initial visit because it can help to uncover other medical problems that may be causing symptoms of a reversible dementia.

Another essential area of investigation is a functional assessment. A physician does this by asking questions about basic, everyday activities such:

- Using the phone, writing checks, paying bills.
- Shopping for food, cooking, eating.
- Bathing, dressing.
- Driving or using public transportation.
- Compliance with a medication schedule.

Clinicians can usually determine a person's ability to live alone after evaluating the answers. Moreover, they often suggest that a family member keep a diary of the person's symptoms and behavior over a period of time to keep track of any changes.

After examining the results of all tests and studies, and ruling out other dementias, clinicians can then determine with some measure of certainty whether or not a patient has Alzheimer's. There are numerous conditions that are treatable or reversible, yet cause dementia-like symptoms. Some prominent examples are depression (Chapter 2.) nutritional deficiencies, metabolic changes, drug interactions and their side effects.

At first, families usually deny that their loved one could have a dementing illness. More important, individuals with the disorder generally dismiss the view that their memory problems need to be investigated by a clinician. They offer countless plausible reasons why the lapses are benign.

It is confusing and frightening for both the patient and the family to admit that forgetfulness could signal something as dreadful as AD. It is much more reassuring to blame events or people for a faulty memory or an ineffectual groping for words. In his compelling book, The Forgetting, David Shenk suggests that denial has a significant purpose. He writes, "denial is an important part of the Alzheimer's experience, very commonly employed as symptoms first appear, or at the time of diagnosis, or at any juncture where a truth is so horrifying that the most emotionally healthy choice is to pretend that it does not exist. The poisonous reality is pushed back into the recesses of the mind and only slowly, in small drips, is it allowed to seep back into consciousness." Denial may be a part of the time of transition that allows people to develop coping mechanisms.

Gary had always been very protective of his wife of 43 years. He's troubled, now, by Paula's behavior. She has been increasingly forgetful and passive for several months. She no longer cooks and he has seen her stare blankly at the test pattern on the TV late at night. Though they have attended the same church for several years, one recent Sunday in the middle of the service, she turned to Gary and asked "where are we?" Gary's brother has known for some time that there is something wrong and he has urged Gary to seek a medical consultation.

"She could have something like Alzheimer's, you know, Gary", he said. "Ah, Paula's just tired lately. Besides, she's always been afraid of doctors and what's more, I heard that sometimes when people get that diagnosis, they go into a tailspin! I'm not going to go looking for trouble" Gary replied.

The natural inclination is to protect a loved one. However, the longer the diagnosis is postponed and treatment deferred, the more one's intellectual and social skills deteriorate. While there is no current treatment that halts or reverses AD, there are medications that may help to slow the advancement of some symptoms when the patient is in the early stages. Furthermore, there are drugs, strategies, and interventions proven be helpful in managing certain behavioral traits such as wandering, anxiety, agitation and sleeplessness. Although an unfavorable diagnosis is extremely difficult for any patient to hear and accept, not knowing what is wrong heightens fear and increases the social isolation for both patient and caregiver.

Health researchers are aware of the reluctance of some people to see a doctor because of bewildering and frightening symptoms. Therefore, more comfortable alternatives are being investigated. The medical literature has described some automated systems used to manage special situations where personal contact between physician and patient is not feasible. The researchers investigated various technologies including interviewing by means of a voice-driven, computerized telephone system which could be accessed by a toll-free number. The system is equipped to identify callers who seem to have early symptoms of AD, dementia, or depression and provides information and referrals to local resources. The results indicate that this seems to be a practical and cost-effective screening method in selected situations.

Technology holds the promise of additional effective tools to add to the armament of clinicians. Nevertheless, there is no substitute for a face-to-face diagnostic evaluation. The first step in learning why a person is experiencing cognitive and behavioral changes remains the personal visit with a clinician. In the meantime, patients and families can do something constructive by documenting symptoms over a period of time in a journal in order to help the clinician more fully understand the person's illness.

The diagnosis of AD can only be positively confirmed upon autopsy. Nevertheless, there are many tests and scans that do help to rule out other possible causes of dementia such as strokes, thyroid disorders and vitamin B12 deficiency. These practical measures often identify the reversible causes of dementia and once reversible dementia is ruled out, clinicians can arrive at the highly probable diagnosis of AD.

Research done by scientists from the University of Pennsylvania School of Medicine has resulted in the development of a urine test that detects chemical damage in the brains of persons with mild cognitive impairment (MCI), a recognised precursor to Alzheimer's disease. The test measures a substance called isoprostane, a fatty acid formed as a result of free radical damage in the brain. The impairment correlates with a clinical diagnosis of Alzheimer's disease.

Although the test is not yet widely available, Domenico Pratico_, assistant professor in Penn's Department of Pharmacology, pointed out that it is the first non-invasive test for AD and would enable physicians to slow the course of the disease if it is recognized early enough. Dr. Pratico_ and his colleagues published the study's results in the June, 2002 edition of Archives of Neurology.

Again, there are compelling advantages to obtaining an early diagnosis. Primarily, an early diagnosis gives patients the opportunity to try existing treatments and it allows them and their families more time to develop their plans for the future.

Stages of AD

Physicians usually refer to Alzheimer's disease as occurring in three stages: mild, moderate and late, or end-stage AD. Table 3.1 describes the three stages.

stage:		symptoms:
First	early AD	Chief complaint is recent loss of memory, e.g., where things are, recalling the right word or a person's name. Unable to learn and retain new information. Confused. May become emotionally unstable.
Second	intermediate AD	May need help dressing, bathing, toileting. Has lost sense of time and place. Gets lost at home. High risk for falls.
Third	late and end-stage AD	Unable to walk, incontinent, long term and recent memory lost. Totally dependent. Possible seizure activity. At risk for infections.

Table 3.1.

There is wide variation in the way the disease affects patients. The common characteristic is cognitive decline, but the rate at which it advances is uneven. Generally, survival ranges from 2 to 20 years, with an average of 7 years.

RISK FACTORS

Most information about Alzheimer's disease refers to three major risk factors, none of which can be modified: gender, age and family history. Although women appear to have a somewhat higher rate of Alzheimer's than men, this is probably not due to a biological factor but rather to their greater longevity.

note

Age estimates of prevalence of AD ***65 - 74*** *1 in 26,* ***75 - 84*** *1 in 6,* ***85+*** *1 in 2*

However, there are two equally significant factors that can be modified: hypertension and elevated serum cholesterol in a middle aged (about 50) person. (see p. 19)

Mild cognitive impairment (MCI), a borderline condition between normal, age-related memory loss and early AD, is a risk state for AD. While it is an memory impairment that is associated with a more serious problem, some clinicians object to the term MCI claiming it is non-specific and leads to generalization. Nonetheless, all agree that MCI usually heralds dementia of the Alzheimer type. Persons diagnosed with MCI are followed closely by their physicians and who test their cognitive abilities such as language, reading, writing, reasoning and understanding. Imaging studies done at this stage may show atrophy of the hippocampus, (see fig. 3.2 C.) an important change that can predict cognitive impairment. Drugs approved to delay AD onset, e.g., donepezil, rivastigmine and galantamine may be used at this time.

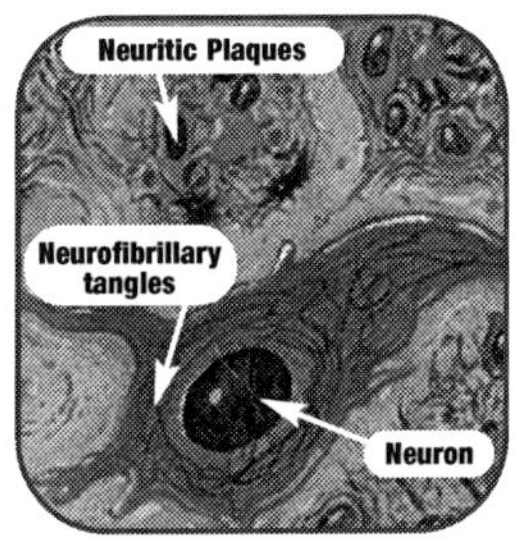

Source: Institute of Neurologic Disorders and Stroke, National Institutes of Health. www.ninds.nih.gov/index

Figure 3.1 Illustration showing hallmarks of Alzheimer's disease include neuritic plaques, (outside neurons), and neurofibrillary tangles (inside neurons).

A. **Cerebral Cortex:**
Involved in conscious thought and language.

B. **Basal forebrain:**
Has large numbers of neurons containing acetylcholine, a chemical important in memory and learning.

C. **Hippocampus:**
essential to memory storage

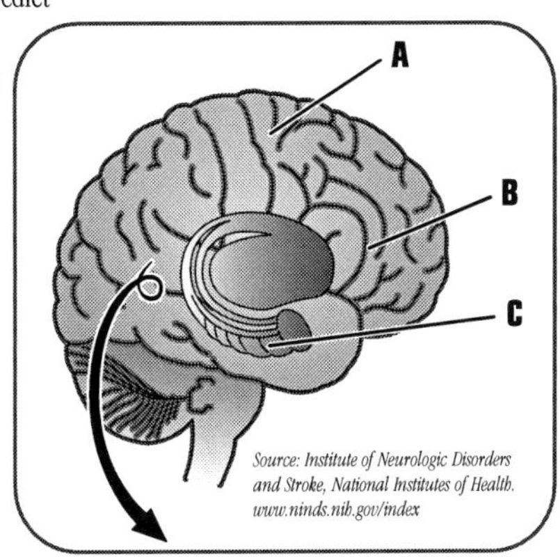

Figure 3.2 illustration of brain (cortex, forebrain, hippocampus)

Hypertension / Elevated Blood Cholesterol

A study done in Finland and published in 2001 in the British Medical Journal concluded that participants who had high cholesterol levels or elevated systolic blood pressure in middle age were almost twice as likely to develop Alzheimer's disease. Individuals who had both hypertension and high cholesterol levels had 3.5 times the risk of developing the disease. It is helpful to know that these are two risk factors that can be modified when acceptable cholesterol levels and blood pressure are achieved.

Some other risk factors associated with Alzheimer's disease are:

- Environmental toxins
- Genetic defects or genetic predisposition
- Down syndrome
- Estrogen deficiency
- Head injury
- Cell death caused by viral or infectious agents
- Medication side effects

All the above risks are currently under investigation. However, many older adults and their families can act independently to reduce the hazards of the last risk factor, the side effects of medications, by learning how and why drugs can be hazardous.

The most common cause of disorientation, confusion and forgetfulness in the elderly is drug intoxication due to <u>polypharmacy</u> – the concurrent use of several medications. People 65 and older consume more prescription and over-the-counter medications than any other age group, primarily, because they have at least one chronic illness, and most of them have two or more.

While no one would dispute that many older adults owe their health (and in some cases, their lives) to new and improved medicines and vaccines, using these drugs can be precarious when several of them are used at one time. Normal aging processes cause physiological changes that often make the aged more susceptible to adverse side effects and drug-drug interactions. As examples, the diminishing liver and kidney functions of older adults means that medications take longer to clear out of their systems when compared to those of middle aged or younger adults.

The nervous system, however, is the first system to go awry when a drug burden becomes too great. Some clinicians make it a practice to declare experimental 'drug holidays' for patients with confusion by discontinuing <u>all</u> medications for a brief period. Frequently the patient's confusion lifts when this is done. After the drugs are reintroduced, the patient is often able to manage quite well on smaller doses than previously prescribed. Of course, no one should discontinue any medication without a confirmation by the prescribing physician.

Older adults and their caregivers need to understand that the term "drugs" means not only all prescription medications but also all over-the-counter preparations including vitamins and supplements. Physicians often ask their patients to bring all their medicines together in a paper bag so that they may fully understand exactly what the patient is actually taking. This is an effective way to avoid harmful drug interactions.

Other safety precautions that should be adopted in the home are:

- A daily checklist that lists the name of the drug, the physician who prescribed it, the time to take it and the dosage.
- Confirmation that the label on the medication is for the person who takes the drug.
- Taking the exact amount at the time the physician ordered.
- Discarding any drug that has expired.

Furthermore, no one should take medicine prescribed for someone else nor should anyone stop taking a prescription unless their physician agrees.

A visit to a physician is somewhat stressful for most people. It can be difficult to know what questions to ask regarding the chief complaint or any new medications. By preparing a few standard questions before the visit, older adults and their caregivers can develop a clearer plan to simplify the medication regimen, help to save time and prevent errors.

The following questions may be used as a guide:

- What is the name of the drug and why is it prescribed?
- How long it will take the drug to work?
- How should the patient expect to feel after taking the medication?
- What are the side effects? Should they be reported?
- Inquire about alternatives to medications.

A local pharmacy is a valuable though underused resource. Pharmacists are trained to explain prescriptions and to offer suggestions that can make taking medications easier an safer. They will also supply labels in larger, easier to read print and provide containers for drugs that do not have safety caps if people have trouble opening the medicine bottle.

Treatment

Although a diagnosis of AD is devastating to both patient and family, there are treatments that seem to alleviate symptoms. Many people in the early and middle stages of the disease find these measures to be helpful. Furthermore, there are reliable therapies available that can help with the behavioral problems of sleeplessness, wandering, agitation, anxiety and depression. Being able to manage these aspects of the illness is doubly beneficial because it has the dual effect of making the patient more comfortable and easing the burden on their caregivers.

The only drugs currently approved by the U. S. Food and Drug Administration (FDA) to treat AD and which are commonly used internationally are tacrine, donepezil, rivastigmine and galantamine. These drugs act by preserving an essential neurotransmitter, acetylcholine, the chemical which governs the function of brain cells responsible for memory, thought and judgment. However, like all drugs, they have side effects and the potential to interact with other drugs.

A recent Australian clinical trial of a new drug, clioquinol, has had encouraging results. The drug works by reducing plaque in the brain. It does this by dissolving the protein and allowing for its elimination. As a result, the destructive plaque is prevented from accumulating.

Clioquinol appeared to slow the decline of cognitive test scores of the patients involved in the research. Dr. Colin Masters at the University of Melbourne reported the study's results in the Archives of Neurology, December, 2003.

Health care practitioners can refer to: Evidence Based Clinical Practice Guidelines available at **http://www.ncl.ac.uk/chsr/publicn/guide/dementia.pdf**

Source:
University of Newcastle upon Tyne,
NE1 7RU, United Kingdom,
Telephone: (0191) 222 6000
From outside the UK dial +44 191 222 6000

A clinical practice guide to Alzheimer's disease for the consumer is available at:
http://www.ahcpr.gov/clinic/alzcons.htm

The site **www.alzheimer-europe.org** can supply families with practical tips, a care manual, and the latest information on research and medications. It links to related sites.

New research has shown that a vaccine, aimed at preventing or reversing the formation of AD-associated pathologic lesions, might one day be a useful therapy. Recent results using a mouse model suggest that immunological interventions may retard and even reverse the development of some of the pathologic changes associated with AD. Early clinical trials to test the vaccine are still in progress but offer hope for future therapy.

Under Investigation

The implantation of a shunt in the brain to drain off toxic elements in the cerebral spinal fluid is presently being evaluated in a few Alzheimer's patients. Early reports are that the participants showed a stabilization of their thinking skills. However, more research is needed before such surgery is determined to a viable choice for AD patients.

Complementary and alternative medicine

Complementary or alternative medicine also has an important role in the treatment of AD. As an example, vitamin E is a supplement that is part of standard AD therapy. Another widely available natural product is ginko biloba, a mainstay in Chinese herbal medicine for several centuries. However, while this remedy is used extensively in Europe and Asia, researchers in the United States caution that more investigation is needed before it is recommended for general use.

Alternative or complementary therapy is not strictly regulated and consumers need to guard against unscrupulous practitioners. Both patients and caregivers should consider several factors before choosing practices or remedies that have anecdotal but not evidence-based support. For example, makers of herbal supplements often promote the fact that their products are "natural". However, many of these natural products, sold as herbal supplements, alter the action of a prescription or increase the drug's side effects. Countless numbers of herbal remedies are totally useless. Nevertheless, there are ways to determine the safety and effectiveness of the product or treatment, the qualifications of the health care practitioner and the quality of the service delivery. A good place to begin this investigation is at the National Center for Complementary and Alternative Medicine (NCCAM) at the National Institutes of Health. The web site is **www.nccam.nih.gov.** Information is also available from the NCCAM Clearinghouse at:

NCCAM Clearinghouse,
P. O. Box 7923,
Gaithersburg, MD 20898-7923.
1-888-644-6226
Fax: 1-866-464-3616,
TTY: (for the hearing impaired) 1-866-464-3615
e-mail: info@nccam.nih.gov.

For international inquiries, there is a wide range of information about complementary/alternative (traditional) medicine available from the World Health Organization (WHO) at: **http://www.who.int/dsa/cat98/trad8.htm** . Featured are instructions describing legal status, regulatory situations, and research guidelines for herbal medicines and acupuncture.

To access the WHO bulletin listing a systematic review of the prevalence of complementary/ alternative medicine: **http://www.who.int/bulletin/pdf/2000/issue2/bu0143.pdf**

Clinical Trials

Patients and caregivers often have questions about participating in a clinical trial for a particular therapy under development. A clinical trial is a research study designed to answer specific questions about new therapies or new ways of using existing treatments. Such studies are done to learn whether new drugs or treatments are safe and effective.

The National Institutes of Health, through its National Library of Medicine, has developed a website **http://clinicaltrials.gov** to provide patients, family members and the general public current information about clinical research studies. For more information about the suitability of a certain person for a clinical trial, call 1-800-272-3900. Two drugs presently in clinical trials for AD are ALCAR and *Huperzine A*.

ALCAR (acetyl-l-carnitine HCL) acts to lessen Alzheimer's symptoms and reduce cognitive deterioration. *Huperzine A* is a traditional Chinese herbal remedy that acts to enhance memory and it seems to have a dual action. It not only guards the neurotransmitter, acetylcholine, but it also may have neuroprotective effects.

ALCAR is not yet approved by the FDA but *Huperzine A* is sold as a nutritional supplement. As with any drug, consult a physician before taking anything not specifically prescribed.

Family Matters

Most people postpone making serious legal and financial decisions for as long as they can. However, as soon as there is a diagnosis of AD, legal and financial planning should begin in earnest so patients and families can make their decisions together. This is especially important if the person with Alzheimer's still has the capacity to manage his own legal and financial affairs.

The following are useful websites that can answer questions and supply resources for AD patients and their families:

- From the Alzheimer's Association's Caregiver's Guide:
  www.alz.org/caregiver/guide/legal
- Fact sheet from the Administration on Aging defining the legal rights of older adults:
  www.aoa.gov/Factsheets/rights.html
- Legal assistance developers refer persons in need of help to the appropriate legal providers for the elderly. These free services direct people to the services they need:
  www.aoa.gov/aoa/pages/lsdevs.html

In a bygone era, families stayed fairly close together, if not in the same neighborhood, at least in the same state or region of the country. Those days are long gone and many adult children are currently facing the responsibility of providing long distance care for their aging parents.

The role of the long distance caregiver is time consuming and stressful, however, there are resources and support available .

Through the Older Americans Act in the US, state and local resources, a network of state and local agencies on aging can provide guidance and direction for older adults and caregivers. The National Institute on Aging's Alzheimer's Disease Education and Referral Center (ADEAR Center) is a public organization that provides information and assistance to families affected by Alzheimer's disease, **www.alzheimers.org/ir/html.**

The ADEAR Center was established by the National Institute on Aging in 1990 to provide information about AD, its affect on families and health professionals and research into possible causes and cures. The toll free telephone number 1-800-438-4380 connects to an information specialist who will help individuals in the following ways:

- Answer general questions about AD.
- Direct queries for information about the latest research on AD.
- Provide information about clinical trials of new treatments.
- Tell people how to receive publications about AD and related disorders.
- Put caregivers in contact with other groups so they may obtain more information, publications and services.

In the US the Eldercare Locator helps families find service providers and formal caregivers when needed. The web site is: **www.aoa.gov/elderpage/locator.html** This service is funded by the Administration on Aging and has a toll-free number at 1-800-677-1116 that relays information about assistance available in communities across the nation.

Two other US government sites that are helpful in enabling families to contact the agency closest to the person needing care are: 1) **www.aoa.gov/agingsites/state.html** and 2) a link to legal hotlines in 17 states at **www.aoa.gov/legal/hotline.html**

The Alzheimer's Association is a non-profit group that supports families and caregivers of AD patients. The Alzheimer's website at **www.alz.org/chapter** can supply information about the disease and guides to additional tips and resources

Contact the Alzheimer's Disease Society

A site useful for international consumers and professionals is:
http://www.alzheimers.org.uk/content/links.html

More information for families living outside the U. S. can be obtained at:
www.alzheimers.org.uk

or write to:

Gordon House,
10 Greencoat Place,
London, SW1P 1PH
Tel: 0171 3060606
Fax: 0171 3060808

Practical information for all caregivers is available at:
http://www.alzheimer-europe.org/JMA/English/tips_carers.html

Learning about the imminent impact of AD is frightening, overwhelming, and extremely stressful. Nevertheless, information is power. The following suggestions can help to guide families:

- Make a plan for the future. Find out what insurance benefits the older adult is entitled to. Become educated about long term care options and arrange financial and legal documents.
- List questions for the primary physician and inquire about the appropriate treatments to relieve symptoms and manage behavioral problems.
- Learn what caregiver options are available through the Alzheimers Association. (see sites on p.26) Consider joining a support group either in person or online. The members can be very helpful because of their own experiences with the disease.
- Try to develop a daily routine corresponding to the way the patient functions at a particular time of the day.
- Use adult day care or respite services for the person with AD to relieve some of the pressure of the burden of care-giving.

AD patients and their families need to learn all they can about the disease in order to plan ahead and make the decisions and choices that allow them full participation in managing the illness. Both patients and caregivers need to know what to expect and how to prepare for the inevitable changes. The diagnosis of Alzheimer's disease is bleak, but support is widely available and there is promising, accelerated research that offers hope.

CHAPTER 4

Geriatric Mental Illness

By the year 2030, the number of elderly people who will be afflicted with mental illness in the US is estimated to be about 15 million., a figure that could signal the impoverishment of the national health care system.

Not only is the incidence of mental illness more prevalent in today's older adults, scientists have learned that psychiatric illnesses such as depression, anxiety disorders and the less frequent, schizophrenia, seem to be increasing worldwide in the population of individuals born between 1946 and 1964. Researchers warn that the increase also heralds a more serious threat, what some call a demographic time bomb: an increase in Alzheimer's disease in older adults. Whether it's Alzheimer's, schizophrenia, general anxiety disorders, or severe depression, there is no doubt that the US is on the brink of a national crisis in geriatric mental health. The situation is worsening not only because of the increasingly large numbers of older adults with the illnesses but because clinicians, communities and the managed care industry are poorly equipped to deal with the situation.

The World Health Organization (WHO) indicates that the significant changes in the global elderly population results from socio-demographic shifts and advances in sanitation and public health. These are the two main factors driving the challenges to health care workers around the world. WHO warns that the mental health problems among elderly people are frequent, severe, and diverse. Furthermore, most countries do not have the programs, policies or services to meet these needs adequately.

About 20 percent of all adults 55 and older experience a mental illness and these disorders are not part of normal aging. Of special concern are the strong indications that these estimates are conservative since there is evidence that such mental health issues as geriatric alcoholism and suicide in the elderly are underreported. The size of this group with the inevitable chronic conditions and disabilities of old age could easily overwhelm traditional family and governmental responses for help. In the decades to come, managing the health of older adults will be a formidable task since WHO estimates that by 2025, twenty percent of the global population will be elderly.

THE GERIATRIC MENTAL HEALTH CARE CRISIS

Why is geriatric mental health facing such a critical period when there have been so many highly publicized advances in medicine and technology to help people live longer, healthier lives? Although in recent years the development of diagnostic tools and effective therapies for disease has been unprecedented, too many older adults are grappling with life events and mental health problems that are causing them and their families to suffer. As examples, two of the most stressful and unplanned events in a person's life are deteriorating health and the loss of a loved one. Although most elderly adapt to these circumstances by summoning strength and practical help from their families and other social supports, very large numbers of old people are simply left to fend for themselves. These elders can quickly become overwhelmed by situations that disrupt their familiar and comfortable environments thus threatening their security and quality of life. Such stress factors inevitably raise a person's level of tension and anxiety to a threshold consistent with illness. Medical services, community resources, support systems, trained mental health specialists and caregivers are already in short supply, and as the older population rapidly expands, the need for geriatric mental health services will increase proportionately. The system at that point will be unable to service their needs.

A wide variety of mental disorders can affect adults over 65. There are mature persons who experience the development of periodic episodes while others battle chronic, serious mental illnesses all their adult lives. A significant number of elderly are diagnosed with mental disorders for the first time in advanced old age, 80 to 85 and older. The causes are often linked directly to deaths of family members, friends, pets or physical disabilities related to aging. More important, people who live longer also have more opportunity to develop a mental illness in old age that is related to some chronic physical condition such as stroke or diabetes. These can be disorders ranging from the troubling to the deadly, but all of them require effective, appropriate mental health services.

The current burgeoning population of elders aged 85 and older will continue to grow for decades because the average life span has increased so dramatically and this situation will probably strain existing health care systems to the point of bankruptcy.

UNDERTREATMENT OF GERIATRIC MENTAL HEALTH DISORDERS

It is a frustrating fact that many older adults seldom fully utilize available mental health services. The dual burdens of the stigma associated with mental illness and the practice of denying that there even is a problem are two fundamental reasons why mental disorders are undertreated in the elderly. The missed opportunities for treatment are sadly wasteful because there are many strategies suitable for managing geriatric mental disorders and to a large extent, when implemented, they can significantly improve the affected person's quality of life and well-being.

Other reasons older adults underuse mental health services are:

- Misdiagnosis by a health care provider
- Shortage of geriatric mental health personnel, both professional and paraprofessional

- Inadequate funding for mental health services
- Poor collaboration and coordination among primary care clinicians and mental health and geriatric services providers

Gordon, an elderly widower, lived in a senior citizen housing complex. For the last few months each time his son visited, Gordon would repeat stories about the other residents spying on him and listening in on his phone conversations. He accused one neighbor of stealing food from his refrigerator and another of plotting to intercept his mail. When the son tried to reassure Gordon that his fears were groundless, Gordon became red in the face, pounded on the kitchen table and shouted irately at his son.

Catherine has occupied the same second floor apartment in a large city for more than 50 years. When the resident beneath Catherine's apartment complained about water dripping from her kitchen ceiling, the superintendent and a plumber entered Catherine's apartment to find the source of the leak They found her sink clogged and overflowing. But they also found that each room was filled with trash, broken furniture, stacks of newspapers and magazines even discarded packing cartons that the woman had apparently retrieved from a dumpster.

Rita, age 87, lives on a fixed income in a very modest home. She regularly buys magazines from telemarketers targeted for car enthusiasts, pet owners and teens. (Rita has no pets and she has never owned a car.) Her son recently took over the management of her finances and he learned that not only has his mother contributed to every charity that she saw advertised on TV but she recently bought a inappropriate insurance policy. Rita doesn't remember any of the transactions and yet it is with great reluctance she is allowing her son to help her manage her affairs.

SECURING HELP FOR ELDERS IN NEED OF MENTAL HEALTH SERVICES

Although it is clear that Gordon, Catherine and Rita display some of the characteristics of dementia and need treatment, it is in no way certain that they will receive timely and appropriate assistance. By some estimates a mere 50 percent of older adults who admit that they need help for a mental health problem receive any kind of treatment. Furthermore, only a small percentage of that number receive the type of therapy intended for a geriatric population. In the face of such dismal statistics, how can anyone be sure that their loved one will get help when they need it? The first step is to encourage the individual to overome the barriers of denial and stigma and see their primary care physician.

---

note

In the event that a loved one becomes a threat or danger to himself or others, call 911 or the community mental health services.

In the past, the funding of adult mental health services was directed toward costly institutional care. This is no longer the case because of judicial rulings that have eliminated institutionalization except in extreme situations. Today, mental health treatment is most frequently found in community based services. However, it can often be difficult for elderly people to take advantage of these options for the following reasons:

- The growing reliance on managed care (the need for a referral).
- Directing mental health services to specialized groups that exclude the elderly.
- Emphasizing services more for those individuals who are severely and chronically mentally ill and rejecting those with a potentially reversible cognitive impairment or dementia.

Moreover, many community mental health organizations are ill-equipped to meet the mounting physical health needs of older adults. One major obstacle is improving accessibility for elders who need help with transportation or who may have mobility limitations. In spite of the fact that there is a growing need for psychiatric home care services, few states view geriatric mental illness as a priority.

The delivery of mental health services could be improved by increasing public awareness of mental health issues. This can be done by establishing advocacy groups, supporting research in geriatric mental health, improving the preparation of geriatric mental health workers, and developing active partnerships between geriatric care services and mental health systems.

Falls and Dementia

In researching the frequency of falls, a common occurrence in the lives of all older adults, the World Health Organization estimates that every person over 65 suffers at least one fall each year. WHO goes on to warn that such falls are not only more common but that they have many more serious consequences in elderly people than in younger people. Furthermore, WHO reports that the number of people over 85 who fall is about eight times greater than in the age group 65-69. About one-third of those injured suffer fractures as a consequence of their falls

sources of direct costs of fall injuries:
hospital and nursing home fees
physician and other professional services
rehabilitation
community based services
use of medical equipment
prescription drugs
home modifications
insurance administration fees

figure 4.1 sources of direct costs of fall injuries

Everyone who has dementia is at an increased risk for falls and the related consequences of long term disability or death. However, clinicians and their elderly patients are becoming more aware of this growing public health problem and the major financial impact of falls and fall-related injuries. In 1994 the National Center for Injury Prevention and Control in the US revealed that the total direct cost (see figure 4.1) of all fall injuries for people age 65 and older was $20.2 billion. By 2020, the cost of fall injuries in the U. S. is expected reach at least $32.4 billion. The costs in the international community is proportionate.

A fall can signal the end of independent living for an elderly person. The long term consequences of the injuries that older adults sustain because of their falls does not take into account any of the disability or quality of life issues for them and their families.

note

The primary cause of accidental death in older adults is a fall.

DEMENTIA AS A FACTOR IN FALLS

There are many intricate mechanisms in the body that regulate the ability to stay upright and maintain balance. With aging, individuals experience changes in vision, hearing, muscle strength, posture, balance and reaction time all of which increases the risks for falls. In addition, older persons are more likely to have chronic illnesses that can affect their balance, e.g., diabetes, disorders of the heart, blood vessels, nervous system and thyroid gland.

There is a strong link between incontinence and falls. This may be due in part to an unsteady rush to the bathroom in the middle of the night. However, since incontinence is also associated with increasing confusion an affected family member needs to be evaluated for this condition by a physician or nurse. There are many effective solutions to this problem ranging from scheduled toileting and biofeedback to the use of medications, incontinence apparel, and surgery.

Osteoporosis, a disorder seen chiefly in post menopausal women, is another serious condition associated with falls. This illness is characterized by loss of bone mass, a process which then causes bones to become brittle and very easily fractured.

Finally, many of medications elderly individuals take can cause dizziness or lightheadedness. These factors, in conjunction with the structural and neurochemical degeneration that are the consequences of dementing illnesses, contribute to increasing the risk for falls in anyone with dementia.

Falls are caused by both external and internal factors. As examples, a slippery floor is considered an external factor and poor vision is an internal factor. Historically, falls have been called 'accidents'. However, a closer look at the circumstances surrounding the person who falls will usually reveal many correctable features.

Persons with dementia are jeopardized not only by the normal changes of aging but also by the side effects of their medications and the potential hazards of their environments. Periodic visits with the clinician who is treating the older adult with dementia are opportunities to assess that patient for gait and balance problems, foot disorders, weakness of the lower extremities, and vision and hearing deficits.

Evidence exists indicating that the most effective fall prevention strategies include both behavioral and environmental elements. Although falls are common in older adults, there are several safety measures that can be taken to improve a person's stability and to avoid future falls:

- Stairs and hallways should be well lit, free of clutter and have hand rails where needed.
- Bathrooms should have nightlights and grab bars placed both inside and outside of tubs, showers and near toilets.
- Non-skid mats, abrasive strips or carpet should be placed on all surfaces that may get wet.
- Living areas should have electrical cords and telephone wires placed away from the traffic patterns.
- Rugs should be secured to the floor.
- Furniture (especially low coffee tables) and other objects can be arranged so they do not obstruct the normal traffic pattern.
- Couches and chairs should be the proper height to facilitate use.

People with dementia often fall out of bed, so in addition to night lights, families often provide their relative with either a very low bed, or in some situations, a mattress placed directly on the floor.

Another approach to fall prevention includes a change or reduction in medications taken by the person with dementia. This possibility can be discussed with the physician. Exercises that strengthen the lower extremities will improve balance, walking and stairclimbing ability which are important well-being and quality of life issues. Physicians or physical therapists can devise an exercise program that will promote strength and balance in individuals, regardless of age.

A recent large study of falls took place in Australia where three factors were examined as fall preventives: exercise, improving vision and correcting fall-risks in the home. The single most important factor was found by the researchers to be exercise. However, a combination of all three factors decreased the annual fall rate by 14 percent.

MYTHS AND FACTS ABOUT MENTAL FUNCTIONING IN OLD AGE

As mentioned earlier, denial by families of their loved one's memory problems and the haunting shadow of mental illness's stigma are two of the chief reasons why the mental health needs of older adults are not fully met. However, it is important to dispel the misconceptions of some of the well-entrenched myths about brain disorders in elderly persons:

- **myth** - *Intellectual abilities in old people often deteriorate.*

- **fact** - Although some cognitive abilities do decline with age, most show very little change and others may even improve. For example, the rate at which an elderly person processes information slows with aging. Although this is normal, it is probably the reason that older adults learn at a slower rate and why they may require new information or instructions to be repeated to them.

  The ability to find the right word does decline (the tip-of-the-tongue experience) but this does not mean that the words are lost merely that the recall ability lags. Most older adults learn to compensate rather well for this problem by increasing the frequency of their pauses to allow time to retrieve the word they want, or else by using a generic term for the missing word. Generally, language skills in the elderly are well maintained. There is no evidence to indicate that vocabulary is lost. In fact, verbal comprehension and the ability to combine words expressively often increases as people grow older.

- **myth** - *Elderly persons with psychiatric illnesses are senile and therefore untreatable.*

- **fact** - Senility is a counterproductive and particularly offensive term because it perpetuates the false notion that all old people eventually will experience a cognitive decline and it wrongly implies an irreversible condition. Older adults with Alzheimer's disease, dementia or depression all have treatment options. There are presently more promising treatments and strategies than ever before which mental health care providers can offer their patients. The use of individual and group therapy, behavioral care plans and appropriate medications are some of the more effective and practical treatment strategies.

- **myth** - *Memory loss is a part of aging.*

- **fact** - Memory loss and dementia commonly associated with old age are not part of the normal aging process. Although the mind is not a muscle that you can exercise, mental activity is unquestionably the key to strengthening and maintaining brain function. Learning a new skill such as how to use a computer, playing cards, reading widely and participating in word games (see p.14 maintaining intellectual function) are all activities that can help elders to maintain their cognitive abilities. Recent findings strongly imply that most brain malfunction can be attributed to some disease process that is not linked directly with old age. There are many medical reasons that can cause brain cells to malfunction or die and they include certain viral infections, unhealthy behaviors such as chronic alcoholism and substance abuse and disorders of the nervous system such as Alzheimer's disease or a history of transient ischemic attacks called TIA's or mini-strokes.

- **myth** - *Having long lived parents is one of the most important factors in healthy aging.*
- **fact** - Although some destructive genetic diseases and their dismal prognoses still exist, e.g., Huntington's disease, there are many examples of familial conditions that can be successfully treated and even eliminated. More and more people are living longer, healthier lives because they modified the risk factors in their family history for heart disease, certain cancers, and hypertension. Alterations in lifestyle with healthier diets, exercise and prudent medication is the prescription for a healthy old age.
- **myth** - *Persons with Parkinson's disease will develop dementia.*
- **fact** - Although patients who have Parkinson's disease (PD) may be at a slightly increased risk for developing dementia, many do not develop cognitive impairment. However, anti-parkinsonian medications have the potential for causing confusion. If a PD patient develops symptoms of confusion, troubled thinking, or lapses of memory, it may mean that an adjustment in medication is needed. Another well-known reversible cause of dementia is depression which very commonly coexists with Parkinson's disease. When the depression is treated, the symptoms of confusion usually abate.
- **myth** - *Head injury can lead to Alzheimer's disease.*
- **fact** - Research has shown that Alzheimer's disease (AD) is more common among individuals who have sustained a severe head injury accompanied by loss of consciousness. However, it is unclear whether some head trauma is a result of falls during the early stages of AD or whether AD results from an earlier injury to the head. More research is needed to fully understand the link between AD and head injury.

MAINTAINING INTELLECTUAL FUNCTION

There is no diet, pill or herbal remedy that can guarantee healthy brain function through adulthood into old age. However, there is evidence showing that certain factors are associated with strong mental functioning in old age, e.g., participation in regular physical activity, having a solid social support system and having confidence in one's ability to deal with the future.

Commonsense strategies anyone can use to help ensure optimal memory by maintaining a healthy body are:

1. **Eating a healthy diet.** A balanced diet will protect the body from many diseases that can cause brain cells to malfunction or die. The importance of dietary and lifestyle factors cannot be underestimated and two of the most essential goals would be lowering cholesterol and

avoiding smoking. These positive health practices are clearly linked to a smaller percentage of elderly needing help with their activities of daily living.

2. **Participating in regular exercise.** The brain needs oxygen to function and exercise enhances the delivery of oxygen to the brain that is required for it's peak performance. If the arteries that supply the brain with the essential nutrients of oxygen and glucose are obstructed by cholesterol, the circulation to the brain is impaired and brain function diminishes. Exercise also optimizes the immune system thereby increasing the body's ability to resist disease.

3. **Getting a good night's sleep.** Chronic sleep problems should be treated because they are proven health risks. Sleep apnea, for example, in which a person has brief interruptions of breathing while asleep, can impair brain cells as well as cause other serious health problems. The research indicates that treating sleep apnea can reverse dementia in selected patients. Furthermore, elderly people with sleep apnea are found to be more prone to depression.

4. **Staying active mentally.** The benefits of stimulating the brain at all ages cannot be overemphasized. Such pastimes as reading widely, participating in word games, or learning new skills and activities that challenge the mind are all extremely beneficial.

5. **Being aware of drug interactions.** Many medications can cause feelings of disorientation, confusion, fatigue or poor concentration. Physicians need to know all the prescriptions, over-the-counter remedies, vitamins and herbal products their patients consume.

As the number of older adults continues to increase in the 21st century, it is helpful to be aware of the fictions and realities of aging. Elderly individuals and their families who are armed with facts about the developmental and emotional aspects of old age will be more successful in maintaining good physical and mental health.

Psychiatric Treatment of the Geriatric Patient

Some of the warning signs of mental illness are personality changes, persistent sadness, inability to cope with daily activities, suspicious or hostile behavior and the abuse of alcohol or other drugs. Dementia and other mental disorders were once considered the usual and unavoidable consequences of old age and there was little hope or expectation for improvement. However, with the development of diagnostic and therapeutic tools to treat geriatric psychiatric disorders there are now many more opportunities to improve the mental health of older adults, enhance their quality of life and well-being while strengthing family relationships.

More than half of the older adults who need psychiatric treatment seek help first from their primary care physician. There is not the overt perception of stigma when a patient sees a primary care physician for mental health services as there may be when one visits a psychiatrist or a psychologist. Moreover, many insurance policies encourage the initial use of primary care physicians. Often, too, elders find this option more convenient and they may be more comfortable discussing troubling emotional issues with the doctor that they see regularly.

There are certain drawbacks, however. Most primary care physicians are not well trained in the treatment of mental disorders. Consequently, some may mistakenly attribute psychiatric symptoms either to a coexisting physical problem or to the fact that the patient is old. Under these circumstances there is significant risk that although the symptom will be treated, the underlying cause may not be determined. Finally, there are still some physicians who have an age bias that may prevent them from effectively treating their elderly patients.

If the decision is made that medical treatment by a mental health professional is indicated, the patient will be referred to a psychiatrist, i.e., a physician who has spent many years training in the field of medicine dealing with the diagnosis, treatment and prevention of mental illness. Unlike other therapists, the psychiatrist can prescribe appropriate medication.

Geriatric psychiatry is a relatively young branch of medicine. Psychiatrists with this special training focus on the diagnosis and treatment of mental disorders that afflict the elderly, chiefly, anxiety, depression and dementia. Such a clinician understands the specific physical and emotional needs of the aged and is able to develop an effective treatment plan that addresses these needs comprehensively. Moreover, clinicians with these credentials can help to educate families in their caregiver roles while integrating existing medical illnesses, medications and family concerns in the program of care.

The Significance of Mental Illness in Long Term Care

Only in recent years has there been widespread acceptance by health care workers that many cases of mental illness in the nursing home population can be effectively treated. The American Psychiatric Association estimates that about two out of three nursing home residents suffer from some type of dementing illness, with Alzheimer's disease being most prevalent followed by delirium, depression and other chronic conditions that can lead to dementia. Many researchers have suggested that between 80 and 90 percent of long term care residents have some form of psychiatric disorder. Nonetheless, despite the widespread acknowledgment that geriatric mental disorders exist and are treatable, most health care providers agree that the problem still lacks sufficient attention and emphasis.

Leading professionals in geriatric mental health distinguish between mental and physical health care. They decry the practice of simply treating symptoms without looking for the root cause of the problem. As examples, administering sedatives or antipsychotic drugs is not going to help a resident who is increasingly restless and agitated because he has a urinary tract infection, is constipated, or is experiencing pain.

Those working in the health care industry claim that government regulations make it extremely difficult to treat advanced chronic conditions that are not going to get better. Overall, the chief obstacles for suitable therapy seem to be reimbursement problems, the training of staff and maintenance of support personnel.

There are, however, some encouraging signs in several areas of the delivery of mental health services. For example, there is more success in facilities where the individuals with behavioral problems are identified, where staff turnover is minimal and behavioral planning is consistent. Optimal long term care can be provided by using dynamic, comprehensive care plans and by preparing staff to use the intervention strategies consistently as well as administer the appropriate medications

Mental Disorders as They Affect Physical Health

Unless a mental disorder is treated, there is a strong possibility that a coexisting disease may worsen. As mentioned in Chapter 2., depression is a frequently occurring yet readily treatable mental health disorder found in the geriatric population. However, families and older adults alike need to understand how important it is to treat a mental illness since it can have a negative effect on a coexisting physical disorder. A common example is a depressed patient with heart disease. This type of patient will almost certainly experience further cardiac decline if the depression is not treated. Depression and anxiety disorders may affect heart rhythms, increase blood pressure, and alter the blood clotting mechanism. These disorders can also lead to elevated insulin and cholesterol levels. Furthermore, depression or anxiety can result in chronically elevated levels of stress hormones, such as cortisol and adrenaline. As high levels of stress hormones are signaling a "fight or flight" reaction, the body's metabolism is diverted from the type of tissue repair sorely needed in heart disease.

Paul, was an 87 year old nursing home resident who died unexpectedly although he was being treated appropriately for heart failure. The staff noticed for weeks that he seemed increasingly sad and withdrawn, but no mood altering medication was prescribed for him despite several requests to his health care provider for a psychiatric evaluation.

When his personal belongings were being packed for the family, the nurse was shocked to find a cache of his heart medications hidden in his toiletry kit. It seemed clear that Paul's action was as intentional as it was self destructive.

antidepressants

Two of the more frequently prescribed antidepressants are nortriptyline and desipramine. These drugs are better tolerated by older adults because they seem to have fewer and more easily managed side effects. Antidepressants to avoid when treating elderly persons are amitryptyline and imipramine as they can cause a drop in blood pressure which then places the elder at risk for confusion, falls and resulting fractures. Elderly patients are also likely to experience the additional cardiovascular and sedative side effects of these drugs.

Paroxitine and sertraline are selective serotonin reuptake inhibitors (SSRIs), drugs that help to restore the mood boosting neurotransmitter serotonin to normal levels. Some newer antidepressants such as trazodone and bupropion also have fewer side effects than amitryptyline and imipramine and many clinicians prefer these drugs. Patients are more accepting of drugs that have fewer side effects and therefore are apt to be more compliant with the medication regimen. Escitalopram is another SSRI which is used for the treatment of generalized anxiety disorder (GAD), a condition that affects approximately four million Americans and more than twice that number throughout the rest of the world.

There is a newer group of drugs for treating depression called "dual-action" antidepressants (DAA). These are drugs that enhance the supply of two important mood elevating neurotransmitters: serotonin and norepinephrine. Many physicians believe that the double mechanism of action might help the more seriously depressed individual. Examples of DAA's are paroxetine, venlafaxine and mirtazapine. A fourth DAA called duloxetine has long been available in Europe but is not yet fully approved by the Food and Drug Administration in the US.

anxiolytics

Anxiety disorders are characterized by exaggerated and unfounded fears that are often linked with depression. The older adult who has an anxiety disorder frequently behaves erratically and unpredictably, and this type of behavior can be mistaken for psychosis. The drugs of choice for older adults with general anxiety disorders (GAD) are the benzodiazepines ex., alprazolam, oxazepam and lorazepam.

Buspirone hydrochloride is another highly effective antianxiety agent. Buspirone is prescribed in situations where the troubled elderly patient is unable to tolerate the side effects of a benzodiazepine. As is the case with any medication, families and caregivers must let the physician know <u>all</u> the drugs that the patient is taking in order to avoid adverse effects.

electroconvulsive therapy (ECT)

Another useful, yet controversial, treatment for depression in the elderly is electroconvulsive therapy. In the movie *One Flew Over the Cuckoo's Nest* (Kesey, 1975), shock therapy was depicted as a cruel, barbaric procedure. Before the availability of psychotropic drugs ECT was often used indiscriminately in mental institutions to control inappropriate behavior. Patients were not anesthetized, they generally received ECT by force and many sustained injuries because of maltreatment. After the decentralization of mental institutions and the development of a wide range of psychotropic drugs these practices ceased.

Electroconvulsive therapy is often the preferred treatment for depressed elders when the response rates to antidepressant drugs are disappointing or because heart disorders and their related medications preclude the use of antidepressants. As an added benefit, ECT may also be more cost effective than other remedies for the long term treatment of depression. Recent studies suggest that the use of ECT is associated with fewer hospitalizations which also reduces health care costs.

However ECT is not appropriate for all depressed elderly and it must be used with great care. There are inherent dangers associated with seizure activity. Maintenance treatments employing ECT and antidepressants need to be used carefully because of such risk factors as confusion, cognitive deficits, and coexisting medical problems.

To learn exactly what ECT is, how the test is performed, how it feels etc., visit the National Library of Medicine's web site: **www.nlm.nih.gov/**. Click on *Health Information*, then click on *Medline plus*. In the search box, type "electroconvulsive shock therapy". Next, click on *Medline Plus Medical Encyclopedia: Electroconvulsive Shock Therapy.*

Clinicians do not fully understand how ECT works, but they have been aware for some time that certain depressed persons who have had a seizure also have a corresponding improvement in mood. The reasoning is that the seizure changes the brain's chemistry in a way that lifts the depression.

magnet therapy

Transcranial magnetic stimulation (TCM) has been used to evaluate many functions of the brain, e.g., memory, attention, speech and movement. The use of therapeutic magnets is a non-invasive way that seems to improve the moods of some persons with a psychosis or a drug-resistant depression.

Physicians use TCM by placing a powerful magnetic coil (not an ordinary magnet) near the top of the patient's head close to the area of the brain thought to lighten the mood of depressed persons. Researchers theorize that the treatment works by stimulating targeted neurons to perform more effectively. Treatment with magnet therapy is experimental and the long-term effects are not known.

Integrative medicine

Integrative medicine combines conventional and evidence-based complementary and alternative techniques for healing. Physicians who offer these choices to their patients are able to present a broad range of healing philosophies, approaches and treatments.

A therapy is called 'complementary' when it is used in addition to conventional treatments. A treatment is 'alternative' when it is used instead of a conventional treatment. Depending on how they are used, certain therapies can be both. Some examples of complementary and alternative treatments are relaxation techniques, acupuncture, biofeedback, acupressure, massage and vitamins.

Elderly individuals and their caregivers often choose complementary or alternative therapies because they either mistrust prescription drugs or because these options promise a rapid, satisfactory response to a physical or psychological problem. Concerned families, however, searching for the best possible solution for their loved one's problem can be unduly influenced by convincing anecdotal testimonials that seem to guarantee success.

As a precaution, patients and their families are advised to take the time to verify the legitimacy of practitioners and treatments before agreeing to participate in a therapy. The National Center for Complementary and Alternative Medicine (NCCAM) at the National Institutes of Health (NIH) in Bethesda, MD 20892 has as its mission the scientific investigation of complementary and alternative healing practices. The organization supports rigorous research of non-traditional healing modalities and provides this information to the public and healthcare professionals. Responsible caregiving begins with finding out which therapies work, which do not and why. The website is: **www.nccam.nih.gov**. Those without access to a computer can contact the *National Center for Complementary and Alternative Medicine Clearinghouse* at 1-888-644-6626.

The European Herbal Practitioners Association maintains a website that includes many news articles on the state of herbalism in Europe as well as a page of links to more resources: **http://www.users.globalnet.co.uk/~ehpa/**

The decision to use complementary and alternative treatments has significant implications. Before selecting any alternative or complementary therapy, investigate the following:

the safety and effectiveness of the therapy or treatment Do the benefits of the proposed therapy outweigh the risks? A safe product or practice is one that does no harm when used as intended. Consumers need to tell the practitioner about any alternative or conventional treatments or therapies already being used so this information can be used to judge the safety and effectiveness of the total treatment plan. It is also important to ask about risks, side effects, expected results and length of treatment. Patient testimonials alone are are not enough to assess the safety and effectiveness of any alternative therapy.

Controlled, scientific trials and evidenced-based research provide the only reliable information about a therapy's effectiveness.

the expertise and qualifications of the practitioner Look closely into the qualifications of any potential health care professional, whether physician or practitioner of alternative and complementary health care. The practice of complementary and alternative medicine may not be as well regulated in some regions as conventional medicine. Nonetheless, there are state and local medical boards, other health regulatory boards or agencies and consumer affairs departments where information about a practitioner's license, education and accreditationcan be verified. Most types of complementary and alternative practices have national organizations of practitioners that are familiar with legislation, licensing, certification or registration laws. Speak with the practitioner personally in order to learn how information is communicated to patients about methods, possible side effects and potential problems.

the quality of the service delivery There are many issues that surround the quality of service delivery. It is important to clearly understand how the treatment or therapy is given and under what conditions. A major factor to consider is whether the service delivery follows the regulated standards for medical safety and care. This information can be found in the regulatory boards and agencies described in the previous paragraph.

Physicians and pharmacists should be consulted about decisions made to include either complementary or alternative therapy in an individual's plan of care. Supplements, vitamins, botanical remedies and herbal therapies all need to be evaluated for possible interaction with other drugs. Many elderly persons take a wide array of medications prescribed by several different doctors for their physical and mental illnesses. As older adults are typically sensitive to these drugs they frequently experience unnecessary drug side effects and interactions. Since even healthy older adults are known to eliminate drugs more slowly from the body, elders who are ill are still more at risk for drug side effects. All older adults and those close to them – families, friends and caregivers – need to be alert and watch for negative physical and behavioral responses to medication.

Although generally these modalities have not been scientifically proven, the fact that they have been used for generations implies that they may be of some value. Before trying either complementary or alternative treatments, this approach needs to be discussed frankly with the patient's physician.

The following are helpful, informative resources for consumers:

Canadian Mental Health Association
2160 Yonge, 3rd floor - 3e étage
Toronto, ON M4S 2Z3
Tel./Tél.: (416) 484-7750
Fax: (416) 484-4617
Email: national@cmha.ca

http://link.bubl.ac.uk/ISC8941 BUBL LINK Catalogue of selected Internet resources

For a detailed listing of other CMHA Provincial Offices & Regions, please visit CMHA National's web site at **http://www.cmha.ca/english/info_centre/locations.htm**

Other important resources are available at: **http://www.nelmh.org/** which is the National Electronic Library for Mental Health, created and maintained by the Centre for Evidence Based Mental Health, Oxford, UK and **http://www.nimh.nih.gov/** the National Institute of Mental Health (one of the National Institutes of Health) located in the US.

CHAPTER 5

Families and Issues of Aging

As the population ages, more and more baby boomers are struggling to care for their aging parents. The phenomenon of caring for dependent parents is no longer the norm in developed countries particularly since most women entered the labor force. Consequently, few older adults or their children plan for this eventuality. When the need for parental care does occur, the learning curve is steep and along the way adult children experience many acutely painful disappointments, frustrations and failures which are seldom offset by the temporary satisfaction of a few small triumphs and rewards. Furthermore, as both the adult child and dependent parent begin to realize that they have shrinking control over their lives, resentment and frustration can quickly build.

Families soon learn that caring for an elderly parent is not anything like caring for a child. In the natural order of things, we expect children to be dependent on their parents and there is no question that they need adult guidance and supervision. No elderly parent, however, readily relinquishes autonomy to his child, no matter how affectionate the nature of their relationship may be. A few elders eventually may accede with reluctant grace, but most resent any attempt by their children to arbitrarily assume management of their affairs or tell them what is in their best interests.

Dementia presents formidable challenges to caregivers and their loved ones. Aging populations worldwide are struggling with the disorder and its costly personal, social and economic consequences. By some estimates, more than 15 million adults in the US currently provide care to relatives, saving the formal health care system billions of dollars annually. This common situationis repeated in most of the developed world. The majority of caregivers are middle-aged adult children or elderly spouses who are caring for a parent or partner with major functional limitations. It is not unusual, for example, to learn that an 85 year old husband is providing round-the-clock care for his 83 year old wife. Such elderly spouses are in different, but in no less stressful, situations then younger caregivers. They often find themselves at odds with their adult children regarding their caregiving skills and practice.

Harry, 80, was caring for his wife at home after she had a stroke. Eventually he became overwhelmed by the mounting demands of her deteriorating physical condition and he made arrangements to admit her to a nursing home six months before she died. His only daughter became upset that her father did this. She never acknowledged the need for her mother's placement in the nursing home and, consequently, she hasn't spoken to her father in the three years following her mother's death.

When a partner becomes physically impaired or experiences alarming behavioral changes, the elderly spouse may not be able to manage the illness at home, even with professional help. Long term care clearly fills a need and it is an option that often is in the patient's best interests. However, there are individuals who believe that nursing home placement is akin to abandonment. It can be difficult to change these opinions particularly if past family relationships have been poor.

Telling an Elderly Parent That He Needs Help

Regardless of how attentive and loving the adult child may be, older adults dread the thought that one day they might be dependent on their children. Most elders treasure their independence and shrink from admitting to anyone that they need assistance from their children. Others will vehemently deny that they need help of any kind and, furthermore, resent the implication by their children that they do. Devoted adult children may avoid talking openly to their parents about their concerns because the issues are so personal and sensitive. Consequently, it can take the event of a crisis to bring families together in order to discuss whatever the problems are that compromise an elderly person's ability to live independently.

Accordingly, it is possible, and certainly preferable, to anticipate problems and form a tentative plan before a crisis develops. Adult children and their elderly parents can have non-threatening, constructive family discussions about some of the major issues that can limit a person's ability to remain independent before the aging parent encounters serious problems and needs professional help.

Examples of key issues families need to examine together are finances, housing, transportation, health, and legal concerns.

The above suggestions are basic and introductory and families will add many more to the list as suits their individual situations. Adult children can take the initiative by talking about emotional and perhaps, frightening, subjects tactfully and with love. A way to begin is to start with general conversations about health or home maintenance. Questions about parents' elderly friends, relatives or neighbors and how they are managing can lead to natural yet productive conversations. As examples, all older adults have strong opinions about the cost of food, housing and prescriptions so introducing these topics is sure to reveal important and useful information.

Responsible sons and daughters will also watch for indications of diminishing physical or intellectual ability because chronological age alone is an unreliable sign. The following developments signal that an older adults needs to be professionally evaluated:

- Trouble with basic activities of daily life namely, getting dressed, walking, preparing food and eating are situations that must be corrected without delay.
- Poor hygiene caused by infrequent bathing, clothes that are food-stained and inattention to grooming are warning signs to heed and investigate.

topics to discuss:	information to learn:
finances	Estimated current and future financial needs. All government and pension benefits to which they are entitled. Location of insurance policies, names and phone numbers of agents. Location of bank deposits, checking accounts, tax records, name of financial advisor. Location of Social Security number, veterans' service number, safe deposit box and key.
housing	Affordability of current housing. Identification of safety hazards. Practicality of simple home modifications to optimize convenience and safety e.g., improved lighting, railings by stairways, grab bars in bathrooms, widening of doorways to accommodate wheelchairs etc.
transportation	Competence of parents' driving ability. Parents' awareness of alternatives, e.g., mass transportation, senior van service or taxi service.
health	Names of parents' doctors and the medications prescribed. Parents' wishes re. heroic or invasive measures in the event of a terminal illness.
legal concerns	Names and phone numbers of attorneys. Existence and currency of wills. Existence and currency of living will, health care proxy documents. Funeral arrangements, preferences, name of funeral home.

Table 5.1 family discussions.

- Decline in cognitive skills as in getting lost in formerly familiar places, forgetting current information, repeating the same questions over and over, all may be early signs of dementia and require a visit to the primary care physician..
- Health changes such as weight loss, incontinence or unexplained bruises are further reasons to seek medical attention promptly.
- Change in mood. An older adult who is persistently sad, indifferent to overtures of friendship, lives in seclusion or displays argumentative or paranoid behavior needs the help of a mental health professional directly.

Identification of problems in any of the above categories clearly indicates that the affected individual needs help. It is up to the spouse or adult child to find out the reasons why there is a difficulty and then start looking for workable solutions. In some situations it may be enough to contact the various aging networks and resources in the elder's community (see figure 5.1) and help the individual benefit from the advantages of an appropriate program. However, when there are alterations in health or mood, a prompt visit with the primary care physician is the initial action to take.

examples of community resources:
Area Agency on Aging
Meals on Wheels
Senior Centers
Senior Companion Program
Visiting Nurse Association
Telephone Reassurance
Note: Community service numbers are found in a local telephone directory.

Figure 5.1 examples of community resources.

The US Administration on Aging provides a national toll-free service called the Eldercare Locator as well as an online site to help older adults and their caregivers find local services for the elderly. The telephone number is 1-800-677-1116 and an information specialist can help families identify appropriate services in the area where needed. The number operates Monday through Friday from 9AM until 8PM. Eastern time and callers are asked to provide the Eldercare Locator staff with the zip code of the person who needs assistance. The website is **www.eldercare.gov.** and it offers users 24 hour access to community resources that assist seniors.

Another useful US site is **www.benefitscheckup.org.** This is a free, easy-to-use service which identifies federal and state assistance programs for older Americans. The National Council on the Aging created BenefitsCheckUp to help older adults quickly identify programs that may improve the quality of their lives. Many elderly are surprised to learn about the benefits that are available to them regardless of income.

Similar international information is available by using the site of Alzheimer's International at: **http://www.alz.co.uk/**

Additional resources can be found at:
http://www.carersonline.org.uk/carersuk/index.html
and **http://www.buckscc.gov.uk/care_information/directory/money_matters.htm**

Long-Distance Caregivers

In today's world it is very common for family members to be widely scattered geographically. Unlike previous generations where extended families lived in the same neighborhoods, 21st century adult children and their elderly parents commonly live different cities, states and countries. Consequently, many adult children question how they can regularly check on their elderly parent let alone provide elder care without uprooting their parents or abandoning their own lifestyle. Some widely known basic avenues of assistance suitable for all caregivers to learn about are *informal day care services* or senior centers, *emergency response devices and postal alerts:*

Informal day care takes place in senior citizen community centers and churches. This casual system often bridges the gaps between work and retirement, full independence and partial support, good health and manageable chronic conditions for the elderly and their families. Multipurpose senior centers (MSCs) are especially helpful in fulfilling this need. They provide information and assistance about essential sources of community based programs. Many older adults are able to remain independent in their communities because of the availability of certain social and nutritional supports in the following ways:

- Fitness and wellness programs.
- Meal and nutrition programs.
- Transportation services.
- Social and community action opportunities
- Recreational opportunities.

By 2010 the baby boom generation will constitute more than two thirds of the over 50 population. Today's senior centers are adjusting their mission with new and improved methods and systems, e.g., modifying the kinds of interactive information systems and technology-based activities that the boomers currently use to gain time, pursue comfort and achieve access. The senior centers of the future will offer new ways to improve health, relieve caregiver stress and increase the independence of older adults.

Emergency response devices Older adults who live alone can feel safer if they wear a small device such as an alarm bracelet or pendant that can be activated by a simple push-button in case of emergency. This system is also very reassuring for their children. However, caregivers of persons with dementia who are apt to wander need to provide a more secure environment. In the US they are also urged to register that person with a national identity program called Safe Return. This requires completing a simple form and supplying a current photo. In the event someone is missing local law enforcement agencies are notified immediately and photo flyers are faxed to law enforcement personnel and hospitals to aid in the search. A local Alzheimer's chapter can advise families about registering with Safe Return.

Postal Alert Long distance caregivers can arrange with the Post Office to be contacted if the mail carrier notices an accumulation of mail at the address of their elderly parent. There are many mail carriers who know the frail elderly on their route quite well and they assume this responsibility automatically.

Adult children who live far away from their elderly parents always bear a burden of guilt because they cannot visit as often as they would like and cannot spend enough time with their parents when they do visit. This places them in a uniquely difficult and stressful position. Families in this situation can start to organize caregiving strategies by identifying three general areas:

1. List the most important issues.
2. Determine what kind of support is needed.
3. Learn the resources for information and services.

Important Issues Taking an inventory of an elderly parent's home and lifestyle is time well spent. This initial assessment helps the primary caregiver to decide which changes must take place immediately and which adjustments can wait. Prioritizing and planning comes with practice and adult children need to realistically evaluate the ability of an elderly parent to take care of health and financial matters. To illustrate: although both transportation and socialization are important aspects of anyone's life, it is clearly more urgent to get a 93- year-old driver with failing eyesight off the road than it is to arrange socialization opportunities for her.

When considering the environment a parent lives in the practical approach is to look for possible hazards or needed repairs in the home. Determine if the neighborhood is safe and if the heating and electricity are reliable. This is also a good time to learn the names and phone numbers of some nearby neighbors and to leave a contact number with someone in case of an emergency.

Certain obvious physical characteristics are clues to health problems. An unsteady gait, for instance, may indicate dizziness or joint pain, shortness of breath can be due to respiratory or cardiac impairment. Adult children should also take note of any behavior that might indicate a problem with vision, hearing or memory.

The potential caregiver can maximize the time spent with an elderly parent by visiting an adult day care setting or alternative housing location that might be suitable in the future. It is especially useful to go along to a doctor's appointment.. If the family is satisfied that health care is reasonably regular, medications are being taken appropriately, and activities of daily living are performed satisfactorily, the next focus can be on financial and legal functioning. **(See Table 5.1, p.78 family discussions for further topics.)** There is no set formula that ranks the key issues because every older adult's situation is different.

Getting the Needed Support After families determine what kind of assistance is needed they can gather information by using community resources (fig. 5.1, p.79) and the Internet. Many adult children who live a distance from their parents find a geriatric care manager to evaluate the situation comprehensively and draw up care plans to follow as they manage the parent's care. Geriatric care managers are professional practitioners who deliver a broad range of services to older adults through qualified, certified providers. They specialize in coordinating services and managing the many details that are so time consuming for the primary caregivers. Hospital social workers and visiting nurses can refer families to a geriatric care manager. The online resources for this is:

info@caremanager.org, www.caremanager.org/ and **http://www.caremanager.org/gcm/FindManager.htm**

More information can be obtained at:

National Association of Professional Geriatric Care Managers
1604 N. Country Club Road
Tucson, AZ 85716-3102
520-881-8008 (Voice)
520-325-7925 (Fax)

Having a geriatric care manager is not cheaper than nursing home care, but it is an effective way of keeping a frail, elderly person living independently in the community when family members are not able to assume this responsibility.

Resources for Information and Services

The first resource is very likely the elderly individual's primary care physician since an accurate, objective physical assessment can mean the difference between independent living and an alternative living situation. Next, it is also important to learn what community resources are available (see pp.5,6) for older adults. The US Administration on Aging (AoA), www.aoa.gov, has several useful links for older adults and their caregivers.

For those who do not have access to a computer, the address is:
Administration on Aging
330 Independence Avenue, SW
Washington, DC 20201

Telephone:

(800) 677-1116 (Eldercare Locator - to find services for an older person in his or her locality)

(202) 619-7501 (AoA's National Aging Information Center - for technical information and public inquiries)

(202) 401-4541 (Office of the Assistant Secretary for Aging)
(Congressional and Media Inquiries)

FAX: (202) 260-1012

Federal Relay Services - 1-800-877-8339 - toll free relay service to call AoA and other federal agencies from TTY devices-- useful for persons with hearing impairments (off-site)

The website of the US Administration on Aging: **www.aoa.dhhs.gov/network/links.html** displays the many resources of the Aging Network. One of the links is the site for Medicare which also may be reached by phone at 1-800-MEDICARE (633 4227). When calling, a Medicare customer representative will respond. The Medicare website, **www.medicare.gov**, is directly available to provide answers to such commonly asked questions as what to do if a Medicare card is missing, how to evaluate a nursing home, and what the alternatives to nursing homes are. By clicking on Nursing Home Compare, a link displayed on this site, the viewer gains immediate access to detailed information about the performance of every Medicare and Medicaid certified nursing home in the US.

Consumers and caregivers can find assistive technology and rehabilitative equipment through Abledata. This federally funded project provides information on more than 29,000 products available within the United States. Abledata is maintained for the National Institute on Disability and Rehabilitation Research through the US Department of Education and it can be reached at:

Abledata
8630 Fenton Street, Suite 930
Silver Spring, MD 20910
1-800-227-0216

The site at **www.abledata.com** also provides links to national and international listings of disability-related resources.

A directory of international resources is available at:
http://imsersomayores.csic.es/basisbwdocs/direccionesred/directointer.htm and an Internet global primary care guide is available at:
http://www.uib.no/isf/guide/family.htm

Keeping Track of Information

Older adults tend to become high maintenance when they reach their 70's. It takes a great deal of time to keep track of doctors' appointments, medications, medical bills and reimbursements. For adult children helping with money management as well as looking for community resources that will benefit elderly parents, keeping a log is the best way to keep track of information. By developing a simple system and using it consistently one can bring some order to a potentially chaotic situation. As an example, each entry

Tips on telephoning agencies:
Write down key questions before calling.
When contacting any community services, take notes on the application process, waiting lists and fees.
Learn what documents to supply on an elder's behalf.

Figure 5.2 tips on telephoning agencies.

should be dated and a brief description of what transpired recorded. Writing all physicians' names in red makes it easier to reference (since there is always more than one) because they will be seen more readily in a log. In the same journal important phone numbers and useful travel information can be recorded.

In another section of the log a general idea of the older adult's expenses, annual income, net worth, any debts and bank and credit card information can be recorded.

Alternative Living

Today it is rare to find an adult in their 50s, a member of the "sandwich generation", (those caught between children and parents) who does not have an elderly relative living with a chronic illness. Research shows that more than 20 percent of middle-aged households include at least one elderly parent who cannot be left alone and needs help with the activities of daily living. Many of these multigenerational families share living space with their functionally limited elderly parents. Typically, elder care falls to a daughter or daughter-in-law. Yet, as intimidating a decision as intergenerational living may seem, there are rewards to be had in the caretaking role if the husbands are supportive and the children are cooperative. Marital relationships can deepen and children can mature with the pride of knowing how necessary they are to an impaired grandparent.

Many problems can be avoided with frank, timely communication between the older adult and her child:

When Una's 79 year old mother needed hip replacement surgery, Una assumed that she would bring her mother into her home to live. She overlooked the possibility that her mother might prefer an assisted living or retirement community instead. "I was amazed when Mother told me that she would have an aide in her home after the rehab period and then she was considering an assisted living community where some of her friends had moved to after they were widowed."

It can happen that well-intentioned adult children overrate the value of family over the importance of friends and a familiar neighborhood. However, studies show that elders prize their independence and most of them prefer not to live with their children.

Determining the most appropriate living arrangement for an elder can be a daunting task, but it is fundamental to maintaining a high quality of life. Remaining in one's own home is probably the most desired and it even may be the best choice at the time in terms of affordability, the available support system and the physical environment. However, changing circumstances such as the death of a spouse, a disabling illness or financial constraints can precipitate the need for other arrangements and all concerned have to understand that this is a possibility and plan for it.

Examples of alternative living situations are:

- Assisted living
- Congregate living
- Skilled nursing facility
- Adult foster care

Assisted living has filled the gap for many elders who need a level of care somewhere between congregate housing and a skilled nursing facility. Elderly persons who are experiencing mild memory problems, or who have moderate physical impairments and need some personal care assistance in a home-like setting often find that the environment of assisted living meets their needs. More information is available online at **www.aoa.gov/Housing/al.html** or by contacting:

Assisted Living Facilities Association of America
9401 Lee Highway, Suite 402
Fairfax, VA 22031
703-691-8100

Congregate living or shared housing is an arrangement in which two or more unrelated people share a house or an apartment. It occurs informally and also may evolve through the guidance of an agency.

Skilled nursing facility, as defined in the US by Medicare, is a setting for the type of health care that must be given or supervised by registered nurses. Some examples of skilled nursing care are intravenous injections, tube feedings, and sterile dressings for wound care. For more definitions, log on to www.medicare.gov and then click on **Glossary**.

Another important number for families to record is the Medicare hotline at 1-800-638-6833.

Adult foster care or Board and Care Homes are group living arrangements designed to meet the needs of people who cannot live independently, but who do not require nursing home services. These homes offer a wider range of services than independent living options. Most provide help with some of the activities of daily living, including eating, walking, bathing, and toileting. In some cases, private long-term care insurance and medical assistance programs will help pay for this type of living arrangement.

Stress of Caregiving

About 5 million family members or friends in the US, and proportionate numbers internationally, are still living at home because someone is making a heroic effort to provide the required support and assistance. Families have always been the mainstay for frail elders who need help with daily activities in order to remain in the community. The degree of involvement has remained fairly constant over the years despite geographic separation and other changes in family life. The vast majority of caregivers are women responsible for a disabled parent, yet who are also managing full time jobs and the multiple demands of home and children. Most find themselves in the middle of the conflicting requirements of their families and jobs. Fully 70 percent of the working caregivers have had to rearrange their work schedules, work fewer than normal hours, take unpaid leaves of absence or endure missed opportunities for advancement in order to fulfill their critical role. By some estimates lost wages, benefits, Social Security and retirement income amounts to more than $700,000 per caregiver. Furthermore, as their obligations grow exponentially, adjusting to the mounting pressure and ever increasing responsibilities becomes an exhausting struggle that often results in depression.

How did this complicated situation evolve? A review of the shift in the demographics of the past century provides a large part of the answer. In 1900 the average life expectancy was 47. Today, the average is mid to late sixties, and includes overall more than 630 million older people worldwide. Those over age 80 make up 12 percent of that number.

Although the rising life expectancy in many regions of the world is one of humanity's major achievements, health care professionals recognize that the unprecedented demographic transformation will be a serious challenge to all societies. A recent UN bulletin states that by 2020 the world population aged 60 years and older will exceed one billion and that in the oldest age groups, dementia can reach the astonishing prevalence of 25 percent.

In developed countries (such as the US) an unparalleled situation has occurred, i.e., huge numbers of adult children put between caring for their infirm, elderly parents and the demands of their own half-grown children. Many of these middle aged adults had postponed childbearing until their 30's and while they fully expected to meet the needs of their children they had not anticipated also having to take care of their increasingly frail aged parents.

Elderly spouses caring for a loved one assume an equal if not even more overwhelming burden. In 1999 an article in the Journal of the American Medical Association discussed the increased mortality risks for elderly caregivers that were linked to the stresses they endured while taking care of their infirm partners. The pressure of taking care of an elderly spouse clearly increases the mortality risk of the one assuming the responsibilities for the impaired person's daily functions. This situation not only places a frail caregiver directly in a life threatening position but in many ways exposes the infirm elder to a variety of dangers ranging from elder abuse to infection and malnutrition.

Primary care physicians are in an excellent position to judge whether the elderly caregiver can manage a disabled spouse. After an evaluation of the joint health status of an older couple, both physician and caregiver will have a clearer idea about what will be required to maintain the infirm spouse at home. Some of the most basic inquiries will be about managing the following:

- Heavy lifting and turning; getting the patient in and out of bed
- Frequent changes of bed linen
- The ability to toilet/bathe/feed and provide oral care if necessary
- Skill in administering medication

It is highly likely that an elderly caregiver has some chronic health problems of his own and this situation will almost certainly affect the evaluation.

Getting help with an older parent

The need for respite and support eventually intensifies because most caregivers work outside the home in addition to managing their own active families. In order to reduce the constraints of working and caregiving, the following suggestions can be useful:

1. When faced with a conflict between work and family responsibilities, caregivers should discuss the situation frankly with their employers. There may be the options of flex time, job sharing or schedule adjustment in order to reduce the pressures. Many companies offer resource materials, counseling or training programs and more and more businesses suggest unpaid family leave, a benefit that allows the caregiver time at home and the promise of employment upon return.

2. Older children can be involved in ways that are not overwhelming or intrusive. Their participation in the care of an older adult can range from doing chores and errands to assisting with walks in and out of the home and regular visiting. Young people gain by assuming responsibility, developing confidence and empathy, and giving their parent much needed support.

3. Other family members can be asked to share in caregiving tasks. It is most effective to start with a family conference in order to determine peoples' schedules and to learn what work assignments they will be able to assume. Neighbors, friends, and church groups are other underused resources. Many are able to provide transportation, respite care and help with shopping or minor household repairs.

---

note:
Respite care is provided for under many long term care insurance policies. Check the policy to see if this option is part of an elder's coverage.

When more help is needed

If more help is needed than relatives, friends and neighbors can provide, families need to call community service numbers listed in the telephone directory and contact a local Department of Elder Affairs or Area Agency on Aging (AAA). These offices can supply brochures, direct people to specific services and, in some cases, arrange interviews with a care manager about managing the needs of the elderly relative. As an example, many older adults and their caregivers are unaware of the availability of certain services such as the help of a homemaker or home health aide, home delivered meals, legal assistance, transportation and some home repairs.

Area Agencies on Aging can direct caregivers to other resources for people with limited incomes such as subsidized housing, food stamps, Supplemental Security Income, Medicaid or the Qualified Medicare Beneficiary program. (The latter covers the cost of the Part A and B insurance premiums for low income older adults.)

---

note:
The subject of food stamps as a benefit to elders on a fixed income is covered fully in Chapter 7. Maintaining Wellness.

However, AAA's are not limited to helping only low income seniors. They can also instruct families how to hire home care workers, as well as provide information about home care agencies and volunteer groups.

Elderly people who have minor problems with mobility and self care receive valuable social benefits from senior center programs. Older adults with more advanced mobility problems, serious medical conditions and dementia are often candidates for adult day care. AAA's are able to direct families to these types of programs which offer the dual benefit of socialization for the older adult and respite for the caregiver.

---

note:
When an elderly relative has been hospitalized, a good source for referrals to individual home care workers or home care agencies include hospital social workers and discharge planners.

In other regions, ministries of health and long term care can provide assistance and refer families to appropriate resources. When using **http://www.hc-sc.gs.ca/** Canadian citizens can reach quick links that provide information that is alphabetized according to subject. Other web-based health information can be accessed by using:

http://www.canadian-health-network.ca/customtools/homee.html

In the UK, the National Health Service is reached at: **http://www.doh.gov.uk/index.html**

Another international site linking to a broad base of international consumer affairs and subjects that are health related is: **http://europa.eu.int/comm/health/index_en.html**

Home care personnel and how they help

There is help available to cover most of the situations associated with caring for an older adult at home. When planning to hire a home care worker, families need to determine exactly what the worker's responsibilities are, list them so there is no misunderatanding and clearly indicate who will supervise the worker (see figure 5.2)

title:	duties:	supervisor:
housekeeper, chore worker	basic housework, light cleaning	private employer
homemaker, personal care attendant	provides personal care, meal planning, household management, medication reminders	private employer or agency
companion or live in	provides personal care, light housework, exercise, companionship, medication reminders	private employer or agency
home health aide, certified nurse assistant	provides personal care, help with transfers, walking, exercise; performs household services essential to health care; assists with medications; keeps appropriate records; reports changes in patient's condition to registered nurse or therapist	registered nurse employed by the agency

Figure 5.2 home care workers, their duties and supervisors.

Differences between using an agency and hiring directly

When an elderly person is discharged from a hospital and needs certain skilled services i.e., nursing care, physical therapy, speech or occupational therapy, these services may be paid for by Medicare or other health insurance if they are ordered by the physician. Under these circumstances, an older adult may also be eligible for homemaker home health aide services. At the end of Medicare coverage, families are often able to hire the same aides privately at a much lower rate than a home health agency charges.

It is important to understand the differences between hiring home care help directly and using personnel from a home health agency. Whether families advertise in the newspaper or solicit referrals from satisfied friends, there are specific measures to take that will help to ensure the safety of the elderly individual and competence of the health care worker.

Home care agencies generally employ only bonded, insured workers. In addition, most agencies mandate certain immunizations, health examinations, reference and thorough background checks of their employees. These same agencies also require that their employees know cardiopulmonary resuscitation (CPR).

If the elder has signed a 'do not resuscitate' (DNR) form, be sure to inform the health care worker of the patient's wishes and show her where the form is kept.

The health care worker is paid by the agency and the agency bills the responsible person in the patient's family. Home care agencies have a nurse assess the patient initially to determine needs and develop an appropriate care plan. Key questions to ask:

- Who supervises the worker?
- What is the worker's experience in caring for a dementia patient?
- Who is called if the worker does not come?
- Are there minimum hour requirements?
- What are the fees and what do they cover?
- Is there a sliding fee scale?

When hiring directly, the family member responsible should screen the applicant carefully and ask for identification and references and then take the time to contact the references. During the interview, it is important to discuss fully the patient's needs and limitations as well as the worker's caregiving experience and expectations. Training certificates need to be examined closely particularly if the patient has special needs such as blood pressure monitoring or medication administration. The person doing the interviewing should ask questions about certain basic skills such as giving a bath or shower, caring for dentures and the safe transfer of the patient from bed to wheelchair or from a wheelchair to a car.

Points for the interviewer to remember:

- Explain what is to be done, and how the patient prefers it to be done.
- Be sure that both the family and the home care worker have a clear understanding of responsibilities both to the patient and to each other.

- Tell the worker what the salary is and when it will be paid.
- Inform other family members that the health care worker is there for the patient and not for other family members.

Many families find that live-in help is the more practical solution for the older relative who needs continual help or supervision. There are home care aides who, in exchange for room and board, work for a salary that is much less than that charged by agencies and hourly employees. Inquire of an insurance company about coverage for a full-time home care worker and contact the appropriate governmental agencies to learn about social security taxes, unemployment insurance and workmen's compensation. If these steps in salary withholdings seem too complex to manage, there are accountants and other firms who specialize in doing payrolls and in issuing an employee's check with the required withholdings.

If live-in help meets the patient's needs most satisfactorily, remember also to discuss the subjects of vacations, holidays, absences and lateness as well as the discharge terms when the worker is no longer needed. In order to make the caregiving experience a positive one for an elder, provide the worker with the following before she assumes responsibility for the patient:

- The patient's dietary restrictions and preferences.
- A list of contacts in case of an emergency.
- A review of security precautions.
- All necessary keys.

It is in everyone's best interests to draw up a list of alternative coverage measures i.e., home care agencies, family members and neighbors who can readily substitute can in case the worker becomes ill or is late or absent for any reason. If there is not going to be coverage available for a prolonged period, respite care is another temporary solution to investigate.

Respite care, as applied to home care, refers to an arrangement that provides interim care ranging from a few hours to days or even weeks. It may take place in the home or in a long term care facility thereby freeing the primary caregiver of all patient responsibilities.

It is not possible to anticipate every situation that could occur during the worker's period of employment. With this in mind, it is wise to have frequent, informal meetings with the aide in order to resolve any problems either she or the patient may have with the arrangement. A positive, open position is the most helpful and constructive way to resolve difficulties.

note:

Elderly persons are vulnerable to theft and fraud. No matter who is caring for the patient, a trusted family member needs to protect any private papers and valuables that belong to the elderly individual. Someone must also assume responsibility for mail deliveries and monitor telephone bills for unauthorized calls.

Care at home may not be less expensive than either assisted living or nursing home care but it offers a choice for the at-risk elderly and their families that few other living arrangements can offer.

Family caregiving will be even more common in the future because of shorter lengths of hospital stays, the increased use of outpatient and ambulatory care and the growing aged population, most of whom will spend a longer amount of time with chronic illness. However, the pool of potential caregivers is shrinking because of smaller sized families, an increase in people who do not marry and couples who remain childless. Family caregivers save the health care system billions of dollars yet the great personal cost is still unknown and unacknowledged.

CHAPTER 6

Living Arrangements

Few events distress an older adult more than having to move out of his home because he is no longer able to take care of it. When the adult child or spouse make this decision for an impaired elder, the issue is often compounded by feelings of guilt and anxiety by both parties. However, many times the perceived limitations can be overcome by adapting the home to the disability, and it is well worth trying to make some simple, yet functional changes to improve the physical safety and convenience of the dwelling. Countless families have found that home remodeling can make the decision for an alternative living situation unnecessary.

For older adults with more complex health problems, a professional home evaluation by an occupational therapist can be scheduled before undertaking extensive remodeling. By combining the use of certain community services with a home that has been reconditioned for safety and convenience, impaired older adults can often remain in the homes they have always known.

Home modification and repair

With aging, strength and abilities gradually diminish and physical safety in the home becomes the primary caregiver's first concern. Home modification and repair includes all home alterations that make it easier and safer for older adults to pursue their everyday activities such as bathing, toileting, climbing stairs and entering and exiting the home. Adapting a home to accommodate an elderly individual who has physical limitations and sensory deficits increases both comfort and safety.

According to the US Administration on Aging up to one half of home accidents can be prevented by the modification and repair of homes. Well over half of the older adults in the US live in homes that are more than 20 years old and which were not designed to incorporate today's common safety features. (The figures are even higher in other countries.) Within these older homes, most bathroom fixtures and home furnishings are either too low or too high and few have arm supports.

A general safety check should start with the bathroom, by all accounts the most dangerous room in the house.

There are many other areas in the home where design modifications can help to maintain safe independent living in one's current residence. Some examples are ramps and chairlifts for those who cannot climb stairs and the installation of securely fastened railings on both sides of all stairways for those who can.

problem:	**solution:**
Scalding hazard	Lower water temperature to 120°F or less
Difficulty getting in and out of shower	Install grab bars, use transfer bench
Slippery floors	Have all floor surfaces made non-slip
Inability to manage faucets or doorknobs	Replace with lever handles
Impaired vision	Upgrade lighting, install nightlights

Table 6.1 maintaining bathroom safety.

The home of an older adult needs to be inspected for adequate lighting and the resident's vision should be checked regularly. The changes in visual acuity that are associated with aging e.g., the ability to differentiate among small details, are intensified by poor lighting. This commonly shows up as problems with glare and with printed materials. Older adults take longer to recover normal vision when subjected to glare and they may not be able to read fine print. These commonsense measures can enhance the home and eliminate potential safety hazards.

note: other hazards of poor visual acuity
Impaired visual acuity may also mean that an older adult needs help with ordinary activities of daily living and also that he cannot read important warnings or instructions.

Uncorrected problems with glare recovery will make driving hazardous.

Falls and older adults

Most falls occur in the home, and the risk of older adults falling increases with age. Each year, thirty percent of adults over the age of 65 sustain a fall. This rate rises to 50 percent in persons over the age of 80.

All older adults are at risk for falls. The elderly with dementia are at even higher risk because of the structural changes that take place in the brain. The cerebral mechanisms that help the body maintain upright an position, balance and locomotion are slowly yet inevitably destroyed. Historically, most falls have been looked at as unavoidable and unpredictable accidents. However, a closer look at both internal and external factors associated with falls reveals that this may not always be the case.

Examples of internal factors are growing old, having a disease or taking any medication that compromises balance and movement.

note: classifications of some medications that can cause falls
Long-acting benzodiazepines, Tricyclic antidepressants, Major tranquilizers, Diuretics, Antihypertensives, Anticholinergics.

External causes can be either environmental hazards such as slippery surfaces, poor lighting or high risk behavior e.g., reaching for something that is stored in too high a place or the wearing of inappropriate footwear.

internal factors:	**age-related change:**
visual deficits	Ability to adapt to light and dark slows. Glare increases as result of cataracts. Color sensitivity decreases. Distance-accommodating ability declines.
musculoskeletal limitations	Gait changes, slows. Muscle tone and strength decreases. Awareness of posture, movement, balance and knowledge of position and weight declines.
circulatory impairments	Postural hypotension (low blood pressure occurring when one suddenly gets up from sitting or lying down)

Table 6.2 internal factors and age-related changes that contribute to instability and falls.

Falls are also well known atypical signs of certain serious medical disorders in the elderly, e.g., urinary tract infections, pneumonia and cardiac disease.

note: exercise improves mobility
Older adults who are medically approved can enroll in exercise programs that help to build and maintain muscle and bone strength. This type of training also improves balance and flexibility.

If, despite home modification and the use of community services, an elderly individual needs more help, families may choose an alternative living situation to best meet his needs. Nevertheless, that determination does not mean that the older adult is excluded from the process.

Any older adult who must relocate should participate in all decisions to the fullest degree possible and, although all moves are disruptive, those concerned need to understand that the positive aspects can, in time, outweigh the drawbacks.

The most suitable living arrangements are those that are selected after a thorough investigation of all possibilities and an objective consideration of the advantages and disadvantages. Ultimately, a more functional setting has the valuable added benefits of reducing stress for the caregiver as well as increasing the comfort and well-being of the older adult.

Many caregivers have assumed their weighty responsibilities gradually. They usually begin by helping with home maintenance, assisting with financial matters or monitoring certain health conditions. Others tell of being plunged abruptly into the turmoil of full-time caregiving because of a catastrophic event, e.g., having to step in when a parent fractures a hip or suffers a disabling stroke. Regardless of how the decision is made that an alternative living situation is now required, few caregivers are fully prepared to negotiate the circuitous path to that destination. Along the way, there are personal emotions to be dealt with, family pressures to be managed and explorations in an ever increasingly cumbersome bureaucracy.

The hallmark of a successful outcome is sensitivity to the elderly relative's need to feel that he is a respected partner in the search for alternative housing. Having said that, there are still many situations in which the primary caregiver has to act independently on the older individual's behalf. This is much more commonly the case when the person involved has dementia.

Late life decisions

Physical and social changes drive most of the decisions elders make in late life. Their age-related diminishing strength and mobility combined with sensory deficits in hearing and vision can often increase their social isolation. Aging is defined by change and loss and as people grow older they are more conscious of their mortality. Contemporaries - both friends and relatives - die. Familiar neighborhoods are changed and the popular culture seems almost impossible to understand. Consequently, more elderly individuals depend on their families to help them feel grounded and to meet other physical and emotional needs.

In a very broad sense, there are three general lifestyle approaches available to older adults who are coping with the many frailties of old age:

1. Aging in place
2. Living with a relative,
3. Participating in some form of long term care.

aging in place

The term "aging in place" simply refers to the older adult who continues to live where he has always lived. Despite enduring serious disabilities and chronic illnesses, many elders do not relocate to a professional healthcare environment. Fewer than 5 percent of the elderly worldwide live in long term care facilities. They manage to maintain their independence by using community services and the informal support systems formed by family, friends and neighbors in order to remain in their own homes.

"Aging in place" is also marketing terminology used in the senior housing industry to describe lifecare communities. The industry has organized the entire spectrum of retirement from independent living, through assisted living accomodations and skilled nursing in one, large total care complex. They target a mature population with a variety of features to meet fully all their changing lifestyle requirements as they age in place.

Because of today's longer life expectancies, retirees who sell their houses when they are in their early 60's need to consider their prospective requirements for the next ten to twenty years before changing locations. Unfortunately, most older adults postpone seriously exploring housing alternatives until a crisis occurs or they are no longer able to live independently.

The Eldercare locator service in the US (1-800-677-1116) provides callers with local information on assisted living communities and skilled nursing facilities.

International resources can be found at:
http://dmoz.org/Health/Senior_Health/Assisted_Living/Facilities/Europe/
http://www.assistedlivingonline.com/default.htm

More information for families living outside the U.S. can be obtained at:
www.alzheimers.org.uk

or by writing to:

Gordon House
10 Greencoat Place
London SW1P 1PH

These sites link to other sources of information that can be beneficial to families seeking ways to ensure the health, stability and enhanced quality of life of their elderly relatives.

living with a relative

Most adult children feel quite a strong sense of family obligation and that emotion can easily override reason as the deciding factor for taking an impaired elderly parent into their own home. Well-intentioned family caregivers may feel that merging households is not only the 'right' decision but it is often the only arrangement they will consider. The strong emotional ties shared by adult children and their parents are often responsible for the reflexive inviting of an elderly parent to share their homes. As caregivers they are convinced it is the optimum choice, particularly when dementia has robbed their parent of the ability to manage the routine activities of daily living: matters involving personal hygiene, dressing, eating etc. But before decreeing that care in one's home is non-negotiable, the impact on the caregiver's lifestyle as well as that of spouse and children needs to be thoughtfully evaluated. Some preliminary questions to answer are:

- How do the other members of the family feel about a relative with dementia moving into the home? Will they have responsibilities for this person?
- How will work and school schedules be affected by this move?
- What provisions for privacy can be made for the older adult?
- How will the environmental safety of the elder be assured? (e.g., prevention of falls, wandering, and the chance of sustaining injuries in kitchen and bathroom)
- How will the move increase or decrease the stress of the primary caregiver?
- What other alternative living arrangements could be considered?
- Is the decision driven by guilt, obligation or emotion? Or is it a rational, objective conclusion reached after considering alternatives?

If intergenerational living is agreed to by all, it is still wise to have other housing options in reserve just in case things do not work out as everyone had hoped. Differences in lifestyles and mounting financial responsibilities can derail the most carefully constructed plans. In order to avoid anyone's unhappiness when families are merged, everyone needs to know that different arrangements are possible if the new situation becomes unworkable.

When Tina's mother became ill in Texas and needed surgery, Tina took a four week leave from her job. The surgery was successful, but her mother was clearly not the same outgoing, decisive person she had been. Tina didn't know if her personality changes were caused by a slight stroke or if they were a reaction to the after effects of anesthesia.

She saw that her mother was forgetful, unsteady at times and seemed to have poor judgment. Tina immediately realized that she couldn't leave her mother alone in a distant state. "I knew I had a limited period of time in which to get Mom settled nearer to me in Boston. It meant convincing her of the need to move, selling her car and finding her an appropriate place to live. The time pressure for all the decisions was pretty intense. Finally, I just sold the car and shipped everything to a warehouse in my area. I then booked our flights home and kept her with me until I could set her up in her own place. That's what she wanted, and I really felt it would be best for her, too. Right now she's in an assisted living facility. I have an aide with her two hours a day in the morning and I see her each evening. Her lunch and dinner are provided and she has participated in a few of the activities offered. There are certain social advantages. Of course, it's only been a couple of months, now, but when she needs more supervision then I'll make different arrangements."

When 63 year old Sharon's father developed dementia as part of his struggle with Parkinson's disease, she unhesitatingly took him into her home. "I'm retired and I live alone. Dad and I have always been close and he was quite willing to move in here, so the move seemed logical. However, I couldn't manage this situation if it weren't for adult day care. Five days a week my father is picked up in the morning and taken to a center where he is well looked after until he is driven home to me at 4PM. Of course, I am still trying to learn what Medicare provides, what his health insurance covers, what veterans' and pension benefits he is entitled to and what we have to pay for. So far, we have avoided a major health problem but I have no illusions. I know there will come a time when there will be a hospital or nursing home admission to deal with and more red tape to wade through."

When Clarence turned 78 he decided to move into a nursing home as a private paying resident. At first, his few friends thought it was a mistake. In their view he was still independent and there were no limiting health problems that they could see. But Clarence had vivid memories of years spent caring for his mother before he was compelled to place her in a nursing home. Privately, he feared he was developing the same kind of dementing illness she had. Clarence never told anyone how hard he fought to remember the names of his friends and neighbors. He had reminders and post-it notes everywhere in his apartment and he stopped driving because twice he had gotten hopelessly lost.. As a single man with no family, he decided that his small savings would enable him to spend a few comfortable, stress-free years in a modern facility and then his needs would be provided for through Medicaid.

---

note:

Medicare is a US government health insurance program for people 65 and older. In certain situations, younger persons with specific disabilities also qualify for the same benefits.

Medicaid is another US government program that helps particular individuals with low incomes and limited resources to qualify for help with medical costs.

Tina's mother managed to live alone for about six months until her aide explained that the mother's tendency to wander and increasing forgetfulness made it too risky to ever leave her alone. She was frequently incontinent and often forgot to eat her lunch or dinner. It was clear that she needed full-time care. Tina was overwhelmed with responsibilities at home and at work and reluctantly placed her mother in a nearby nursing home.

Sharon's father began hallucinating and acting aggressively. He experienced frequent falls and was so confused that eventually she could not manage him in her home. The adult day care manager explained that he needed more care than they at the day care center were able to provide. She helped Sharon arrange the transition to a nursing home for her dad.

Clarence's suspicions proved correct. He not only showed rapid, progressive symptoms of dementia, but within the year, he sustained a stroke and required skilled nursing care.

There are many times when it is just not possible for an impaired elder to live in the same home as his adult child especially when there are grandchildren in the same environment. The older adult with dementia presents special difficulties to care for at home particularly when he is healthy in other respects. Certain behaviors can be alarming, i.e. the outbursts of anger or frustration which may be related to the helplessness and depression the elder feels about his situation or to increasing brain damage.

There is also the confounding shock and dismay that adult children experience when an aged parent refuses to modify high risk behavior. As common examples are the visually impaired individual who persists in driving, or the elderly widow on a fixed income who contributes money she can ill afford to every appeal she receives.

As the primary caregiver, the adult child faces the challenge of striking a balance between maintaining his parent's dignity and independence yet at the same time ensuring safety for all in the household. Before any housing choice is made all parties concerned need to examine carefully the older adult's present requirements and try to anticipate how they may change in the future.

Overview of long term care

Despite public perception, most older adults live independently. Five percent or fewer are in nursing homes. Yet, caregivers of elderly dementia patients need special kinds of help so that their impaired elderly relatives can maintain a state of independence while they try to meet family and job responsibilities.

The phrase "long term care" refers to the entire spectrum of assistance and it ranges from the minimal support given by family, friends or a home health aide to admitting someone into a traditional nursing home and 24 hour a day skilled care. For individuals who are disabled to the point of requiring daily nursing care as well as other support services, nursing homes have the advantage of providing comprehensive care services in a single setting.

Today there are more choices in long term care than ever before. However, for families the key to successful long term care is planning and then staying involved in the day to day management on site. Relatives who acquire information in advance understand more clearly what is available and affordable before they are faced with a crisis. Moreover, families find that a good nursing home is reassuring because it offers the affected individual social advantages and safety that provides both pleasure and security, key factors in determining the resident's quality of life.

Information about the many types of services available in communities can be obtained from Area Agencies on Aging and local and state offices of aging. These agencies are listed in the telephone book under "Government".

---

note: examples of community services
Adult day care programs, Meals-on-wheels, Senior companion programs, Transportation services.

Some medical expenses are covered by insurance. The Federal Medicare program and private "Medigap" insurance only offer short-term home health and nursing home benefits. Individuals need to inquire of the Medicaid program about long-term nursing coverage for people who live on a fixed income. Insurance commissions in specific states can answer questions about private long-term care policies and offer suggestions explaining how to buy this complicated insurance. These agencies are also listed in the telephone directory under "Government".

Internationally there are different options and requirements. Some countries have all-inclusive national health services while others have partial coverage and may recommend or even require private health insurance. Citizens and non-citizens alike can address their questions to the departments of public health in the countries in which they reside.

The European Public Health Alliance (EPHA) represents over 80 non-governmental and other not-for-profit organizations working in support of health in Europe. It's web site, **http://www.epha.org/** has links to other European institutions and agencies as well as other countries' health ministries.

At one time the elderly in the US with dementia were cared for either at home or in a nursing home. There were no other choices. Today there is an **adult day care** alternative in the community in addition to two types of residential settings that help to meet the needs of older adults with dementia: **assisted living** and **skilled nursing** facilities.

senior centers/adult day care

Many elders who live independently in the community fulfill their social and recreational needs through informal gatherings of older adults at senior centers. In addition to offering the companionship of their peers, these centers also feature opportunities for the elderly to enjoy low-cost meals, health screenings, and a wide variety of services and activities targeted towards the elderly.

Senior centers serve a dual purpose. They not only supply recreational opportunities but they are also valuable sources of information about several key social programs, e.g.:

- Nutrition information
- Wellness education
- Volunteer opportunities
- Financial services
- Community action opportunities

An essential part of the long term care continuum is adult day care, a service which is also available in the community. Many structured programs for elders with physical or mental impairments are offered in this environment. Participants find social, emotional, and physical health needs met in protective surroundings and caregivers benefit by having a few hours of respite provided by the agency.

Examples of the services provided are:

- Physical, occupational and speech therapy
- Meals and social activities
- Transportation
- Medically related services
- Wellness programs

Caregivers of mentally impaired older adults look at adult day care services from several standpoints. Some of the concerns to be addressed are:

- The type of assessments used determine the range of the older adult's abilities and needs.
- The individualized, dynamic care plan that tracks the progress of an individual.
- Appropriate referrals to other services in the community.
- Clear criteria for termination of service based on the functional status of the participating individual.
- Qualified, experienced staff.

Adult day care has enabled countless caregivers to maintain their jobs, receive help with the physical demands of caregiving and benefit from the welcome, well-deserved respite. The participant gains by being able to receive certain helpful therapies in a comfortable, welcoming environment, taking part in stimulating activities and being able to enjoy the social advantages of being with other older adults.

assisted living

At some point the impaired elder will need more than informal support. The time will come when the help of devoted family and friends and even Meals-on-Wheels and transportation services will not be enough. Assisted living is a residential setting for elders with disabilities. Independence is nurtured in home-like surroundings and personal assistance is available for those who need it.

Most assisted living facilities cannot guarantee that an elderly relative will "age in place" unless they are continuing care communities. As an example, a resident who develops a serious functional impairment such as needing assistance to get out of bed or who exhibits aggressive behavior, may be transferred to a skilled nursing setting. (Residents with significant cognitive impairment are more likely than other residents to move to a nursing home.)

The types of services offered in assisted living facilities are:

- Meal service in a common dining room
- Housekeeping
- Transportation
- Medication management
- Laundry service
- Assistance with bathing, dressing, toileting, walking, eating
- 24 hour security and staff availability
- Access to health and medical services

Characteristics of assisted living communities

Typically, most residents of assisted living communities are single females in their 80's. The dwelling itself may look like anything from a high-rise apartment to a converted Victorian home and the individual units range from single rooms to spacious apartments. Some buildings are free standing and others are part of a complex that allows residents to move from one level of care to another depending on their changing needs and the availability of space.

Assisted living communities are run by both non-profit and for profit companies and families generally pay all costs although some states make financial arrangements for low income elders. Costs vary widely depending on the geographic location. Those that are located in high cost-of - living areas obviously are more expensive than similar facilities in lower cost areas. Other factors affecting price are room size, the degree of impairment and the services needed.

Choosing the right assisted living facility

The level of care provided at an assisted living facility is somewhere between that of congregate housing - a residence that is shared by several elderly persons - and a skilled nursing facility. Some questions to ask of the director of an assisted living community before arranging admission for an elderly relative are:

- What kind of health and personal care support is available?
- Does the organization coordinate health care services for the resident?

- Does a health professional in the setting evaluate the prospective resident for the types of services he needs and is a family member involved in this evaluation?
- What is the frequency of the services and how are they altered as the resident's needs change?
- Will an admission contract be used and if so, does it describe the services (room, board, personal care, supervision etc.) and costs?
- How is resident autonomy and independence provided for?
- Is there a copy of residents' rights and responsibilities?
- What are the opportunities to attend religious services?

---

note: information about relocation choices
www.carepathways.com*, a site developed and maintained by registered nurses.*

---

skilled nursing

Skilled nursing facilities are more commonly known as nursing homes. They provide their residents with 24 hour services and supervision. While most older persons and their families see nursing home care only as a last resort, the Administration on Aging suggests that this may, in fact, be the best setting for disabled persons with multiple problems which require multiple types of services.

Many nursing homes are certified to admit residents under the Medicare and Medicaid programs and consequently must meet certain criteria and maintain federally required standards. It is important to understand the difference. Generally, skilled nursing is available only for a short period of time after hospitalization. Basic nursing care is available for a much longer period of time. If the facility chosen has both types of care then the elder may transfer between levels of care within the facility and not have to transfer out of the nursing home.

Some of the services nursing homes provide are:

- 24 hour skilled medical care for residents who are total care and custodial care for those who are not.
- Specific, prescribed therapies for residents needing rehabilitative treatment.
- Personal care and assistance with activities of daily living for residents with dementia, chronic health and mobility problems.

International information about housing alternatives can be researched at:
http://www.bl.uk/services/information/welfare/issue28/care-ov.html
http://www.doh.gov.uk/caredirect/text/somerset603.htm
http://www.doh.gov.uk/public/raguidea.htm

Characteristics of the nursing home population

A typical nursing home resident is a widowed white female, over 80 and on Medicaid. Most of the residents are physically and/or mentally impaired frail old people, and all receive medical care and rehabilitation to whatever degree required. Elderly women outnumber the men by 3 to 1.

The predominant diagnosis shared by all residents is cardiovascular disease, which includes hypertension and stroke. However, cardiovascular disease is not necessarily the reason families admit their loved ones to a nursing home. Dementia, incontinence, and functional decline are the strongest indicators for the decision. More than half of the residents who are over 85 have an advanced form of dementia.

Virtually all nursing home residents need assistance with at least one activity of daily living - usually bathing- and nearly 80 percent require help with the more complex functions of daily life which require reasoning and judgment such as complying with their medication regimen or using the telephone.

There are about 1.5 million older adults in the US who currently live in nursing homes. However, the numbers of elderly who will need nursing home care in the future are escalating. By the year 2050, the health care industry predicts that the number will double. The three major contributing factors to the soaring numbers of the nursing home population are 1) the increase in life expectancy with 2) the accompanying increase of age-related chronic illnesses and 3) altered family structure.

The effects of the same issues are being felt internationally. In the UK, for example, more than 1.5 million of adults over the age of 60 have personal care difficulties and 545,000 people, more than a third of the group over 60, are residing in nursing and residential care homes. In most of the countries of the EU, care and support for older people is provided by their family members, particularly spouses and daughters. However, even this custom seems to be slowly changing to reflect the US model.

An online care guide is available at: **http://www.careaware.co.uk/aboutus.html**
Other questions about health matters are referred to the National Health Service at:
http://www.nhs.uk/

Choosing the right nursing home

Initially caregivers need to learn if the nursing home is Medicare and Medicaid certified, if the nursing home and the administrator are licensed in the state in which they operate and the results of the most recent state regulatory survey of the facility.

Many families wrongly assume that either their traditional health insurance or Medicare will cover nursing home costs for their impaired elderly relative. The fact is that Medicare pays only for a temporary period of care if the person is admitted to the facility to convalesce after a hospitalization. Medicaid pays for extended nursing home stays if the resident does not have the assets with which to cover the costs. By some estimates, Medicaid underwrites the costs of 75 percent of those who live in nursing homes.

Individuals are responsible for paying for whatever care is not covered by insurance with their personal funds. This emphasizes the importance of verifying the facility's certification. If Medicaid is not accepted, then when a resident's money runs out that individual will be transferred to another facility.

Nursing home placement is usually discussed initially with the elder's physician, and professional advice of this nature is essential. Most physicians are experienced in assisting families with managing the anticipated physical and behavioral changes of the elderly individual with dementia. They can suggest tested courses of action and help with transitions as well as offer continuing support. However, in order to optimize any placement decision and to protect the older adult as much as possible, families need to visit several nursing homes in the area. A checklist that identifies specific, essential factors is invaluable when the time comes to make a decision. Nonetheless, becoming familiar with certain Medicare and Medicaid requirements is an important first step. Relatives need to understand the Medicare criteria for nursing home reimbursement and Medicaid criteria for the individual.

After the primary caregiver understands the application of Medicare/Medicaid criteria, a visit to the website **www.medicare.gov** yields a fully prepared checklist for persons choosing a nursing home. The same site also shows people how to compare the various nursing homes in their areas.

Medicare criteria for nursing home reimbursement:

- The resident requires skilled care.
- Skilled care is provided only after a three day hospital stay for treatment of the same disorder that was treated in the hospital.
- The nursing home is a Medicare approved facility with a registered nurse on duty 24 hours a day.
- The resident occupies a Medicare certified bed.
- The skilled care required can only be obtained in a nursing home.

Medicaid eligibility criteria for an individual resident:

- The resident is 65, or blind, or disabled as defined by the state.
- The resident lives in the state that is providing the Medicaid benefits.
- The care provided by a nursing home is the type of care the resident needs.
- The resident meets the assets and income limits designated by the state.

---

note:

Medicaid varies from state to state. Confirmation of Medicaid eligibility requires contacting a state Medicaid agency.

The eldercare locator at 1-800-677-1116 can direct individuals to the appropriate Medicaid agency.

More consumer information can be found at:

Centers for Medicare and Medicaid Services
7500 Security Boulevard
Baltimore, MD 21244-1850
410-786-3000

The Medicare Rights Center (MRC), a national not-for-profit organization, works to ensure that the elderly and people with disabilities receive good, affordable health care. For answers to Medicare questions write:

Q/A, MRC
1460 Broadway
New York, NY 10036
or visit **www.medicarerights.org.**

Nationally, the average annual cost of care in a skilled nursing facility in the US is now roughly $75,000. This is a major financial burden and yet another compelling reason for individuals to become thoroughly knowledgeable in this area. Meticulous preparation is paramount before selecting a nursing home.

The level of care provided in a skilled nursing facility has increased significantly in the past ten years. Most of them now provide the type of care that was once the mark of hospital nursing: complex, invasive treatments and extensive rehabilitative therapies. The nursing home staff now consists of registered nurses, licensed practical nurses, certified nursing assistants, a house physician and specialized professional support implementing the prescribed corrective therapies.

As examples, specific rehabilitative treatments are administered by the following departments:

- Respiratory therapy
- Speech therapy
- Occupational therapy
- Physical therapy

There are substantial financial consequences to living in a nursing home as evidenced by the addition of more diverse professional staff and their accompanying technologies. The many millions of informal caregivers who maintain their elderly impaired loved ones at home are saving their countries billions of dollars a year because paid home care is the exception, not the rule, for most disabled elderly persons.

---

note: informal caregivers
Spouses (also elderly and in fragile health), Adult children, Relatives, Friends, Neighbors

---

A word about nursing home placement

There are few decisions more guilt-laden for the overstressed caregiver than having to relinquish the dementia patient to a nursing home. However, while the setting is considerably different from being in one's own home, it is better structured to provide the extra care necessary for frail elders with serious impairments. There need be no regrets when families decide to do what is in the patient's best interests. Furthermore, since caregivers of elderly with dementia have a higher rate of physical and emotional illness than other caregivers, it becomes an opportunity to protect their own physical and mental health by being able to lead a more balanced life.

CHAPTER 7

Maintaining wellness: exercise, nutrition and medication safety

It is no surprise to anyone in the fields of healthcare or economics that the coming decades will see the population of older adults soar. The mission to help individuals live longer healthier lives has, for the most part, been very successful. However, the length of years alone is not enough. Efforts must now be now focused on ensuring that the quality of life is the best it possibly can be.

Old age can be lively and exciting for elders. Nevertheless, many of them and their families struggle to cope with difficult life situations, physical disabilities or mental disorders that prevent a full participation in life. Policy makers in the US and abroad report that the cost of this loss of vitality - to elders, their families and their countries - is staggering.

From the Gerontology Research Centre in Stockholm, Wimo and Winblad report that the demographic trends are of great interest since increased age is the most prominent risk factor for dementia. Based on the demographic statistics and forecasts from Eurostat and known age-specific prevalence figures (i.e. in age classes of five years) it is possible to make a rough estimate of the change in dementia prevalence in the EU based on Eurodem figures. Based on these assumptions, the number of demented in the 15 EU countries will increase from about 4 million in 1993 to 4.5 million at the millennium (2000) and to 5.3 million in 2010, an increase by 33 percent.

There is ample evidence that much needless suffering by elderly dementia patients and their families could be avoided if available prevention and treatment resources were more adequately delivered. Exercise, nutrition and medication safety are three of the most critical components needed for enjoying reasonable good health and productivity while aging. Mature adults and their families can all share in the improvements in vigor and independence brought about by adhering to a regular exercise and activity schedule. The quality of a person's diet also plays a major role in preventing or delaying the onset of common chronic diseases. Accordingly, exercise and nutrition coupled with precautions when taking medicine can be a very worthwhile 'prescription' for staying healthy as one grows older.

Why exercise

Anyone not engaged in some form of regular exercise is gradually but unquestionably jeopardizing his health. Exercise has so many positive effects that there is rarely a reason not to be participating routinely in this extraordinarily beneficial activity.

Unfortunately there are too many individuals, both young and old, who have the mistaken impression that old people need more rest, not more physical activity. However, just the opposite is true because inactivity is far more destructive.

note:
The report of the Surgeon General in the US warns that inactivity impairs health and is an independent risk factor for coronary heart disease.

A natural, age-related loss of muscle resulting in decreased strength and an increased risk of disability can not only be moderated but in most cases actually be reversed through regular exercise. Research has repeatedly demonstrated, for example, that resistance training or working with weights results in improving the power and muscle size of older adults, including those of advanced years.

As an important side benefit for working out, there is no surer way to help maintain healthy blood flow, which nourishes and fortifies the brain cells while simultaneously reducing hypertension and lowering cholesterol levels. Moreover, many researchers are also convinced that the increase in circulation to the brain generated by exercise probably protects it just as effectively as it does the heart, lungs and other vital organs. Consequently, it is widely believed that those who exercise may be protecting themselves against the development of dementia.

Although many elderly persons are benefiting from participation in exercise, many more should be. Maintaining adequate muscle size and strength can make the difference between being able to move about independently or becoming increasingly frail and needing someone else to help with the most basic activities of daily living. (It is understood, of course, that no one should attempt to undertake an exercise program without consulting a physician.)

No one can slow the progress of chronological aging but everyone can strive for healthful aging. A sedentary lifestyle contributes to reduced lung capacity, loss of muscle mass and a host of other deficits that are experienced by elderly men and women. Yet, through planned, regular exercise older adults can control and even improve some of the well-known effects of aging and expect the following benefits:

- Expanded lung capacity .
- Increased size of muscle fiber.
- Increased muscular strength.
- Prevention or delay of hypertension, obesity, heart disease, osteoporosis and falls.

Study after study has clearly shown that fitness programs tailored for older adults can not only help to forestall their physical decline but can also foster sound emotional equilibrium. As an example, current research indicates that certain neurotransmitters, those chemical substances in the brain governing our moods or emotions (specifically, serotonin and norepinephrine) are more efficiently regulated and deployed when we exercise. Researchers have known since the 1970s that the body has a natural opioid system which is involved in the control of responses to stress or pain as well as the regulation of the immune system. Although most of us have seen examples of the good exercise does in terms of weight control and fitness, we are less familiar with the hidden benefits of physical activity i.e., the stimulation of endorphin production, those substances that are our natural opioids, and the manufacture of white blood cells, a process that protects us from infection.

There is also mounting evidence suggesting that exercise not only may improve the cognitive abilities of the elderly but may even be responsible for preventing further mental degeneration. Extensive health data from men and women over 65 indicates that those who exercised were significantly less likely to develop dementia or experience a cognitive decline. Precisely why this happens is unclear but many researchers believe that the improved circulation caused by exercise maximizes the blood's capacity to deliver oxygen. Apparently certain areas of the brain, namely those having to do with memory and planning, reap the rich rewards of this increased biochemical activity.

Depression is without question a legitimate response of any patient who receives an unfavorable diagnosis. Individuals who are diagnosed with a dementing disorder are no exception and health care providers anticipate this repercussion when they tell their patients what their symptoms mean. However, no matter how bad the news is, there is no need for people to suffer. Clinicians have several effective medications and other practical treatment strategies which can provide comfort and support for troubled patients and their distressed families.

One of the principle, non-pharmacologic aspects of the standard treatment plan is to encourage a depressed person to participate in some stimulating activities. Clinicians have been convinced for some time that activity provides benefits far beyond physical well-being and a regular program of planned exercise fully meets this criteria. More recently, a team of researchers at Duke University Medical Center disclosed that they were successful in their study of the effects of exercise upon depression. They were able to determine that aerobic exercise not only decreased depression but it significantly improved the cognitive abilities of elderly men and women.

While the obvious physical benefits have always been known, both the medical community and the public found that researchers uncovered several new facts about emotional health and cognitive abilities that were quite remarkable. The research yielded unsuspected and promising new information.

Scientists measured the cognitive abilities of a large number of depressed patients both before and after enrollment in the Duke clinical trial. Those who exercised showed significant reduction in their depression which implied that for many people, exercising was about as effective as medication in treating depression. The improvement in mental abilities, e.g.,memory, attention, concentration, executive functioning (planning and organization), strongly suggested that the mental declines associated with aging may to a large degree be counteracted by exercising.

Overall, health providers and their patients have learned that regular exercise improves physical and emotional health in the following ways:

- By boosting the immune system.
- By enhancing the drug delivery mechanism in the body.
- By providing increased opportunities to socialize.
- By generating feelings of being in control, thereby empowering the patient.

The results of a Canadian study reported in the April, 2002 issue of the Archives of Neurology indicated decreased walking speed as an independent predictor of cognitive impairment in "exceptionally healthy" adults over the age of 65. Researchers determined that those older adults who walk the least are the most likely to decline cognitively. This risk factor, along with a reduction in delayed recall-memory, can help to identify high-risk individuals who stand to benefit from interventions designed to push back the decline before there is a notable loss of memory.

Many clinicians advise increasing physical and mental activities along with the use of drugs in order to slow the effects of dementia associated with AD. The antidepressant action of exercise has proved to be a welcome, non-pharmacologic addition to the clinician's treatment reserve.

Exercise specifics

People often ask if there is there really a significant difference between physical activity and exercise. Generally, any activity or movement of the body will burn calories, even sleeping, but referring to exercise implies an activity that is structured and uses repetitive movements in order to achieve a goal. The goal in this case is to improve or at the very least maintain a level of physical fitness.

All adults need to understand that the inability to do things for oneself does not happen overnight and it does not happen because of aging. However, when it does occur the chances are that inactivity is the primary cause. Some elders reason that they cannot or should not exercise because they have a chronic illness such as arthritis, heart disease, hypertension or diabetes. Yet, health care professionals insist that many of these conditions will improve with exercise and more important, the evidence exists to support their position.

Sedentary elders become deficient in four areas that are key elements of healthy, independent living:

1. Endurance
2. Strength
3. Balance
4. Flexibility

As each of these capacities gradually decreases in the aging body, the likelihood of needing help with basic activities of daily living will inevitably increase as an individual grows older. The accumulation of these minute losses eventually diminish the older adult both physically and emotionally. Yet, as countless numbers of motivated elders have found to their relief and delight, the small gains reached as a result of a commitment to exercise can often have an enormous impact in terms of independence and quality of life.

Seventy one year old Annette's struggle with fibromyalgia and mild cognitive impairment has kept her practically housebound. She could not go out for more than half an hour at a time

type of exercise:	description:	benefits:
Endurance activities (aerobic exercises)	Cardiovascular conditioning to improve heart/lung function.	Supplies muscles with oxygen. Increases stamina. Contributes to delay or prevention of heart disease, stroke, diabetes, colon cancer. Reduces overall death and hospitalization rates.
Strength training	Exercises done by lifting, pulling or pushing weights. An alternative to weights is the use of resistance bands.	Builds muscle. Increases metabolism which helps to normalize weight and blood sugar levels. May help to prevent osteoporosis.
Flexibility	Keeping the body limber through stretches.	Can help with recovery from injury and in injury prevention.
Balance	Achieved by coordinating vision and hearing with the motor response that involves the large muscle groups in the trunk and legs.	Helps to prevent falls, prime cause of fractured hips and other injuries that lead to disability and dependence.

Table 7.1 explanation of exercises.

unless she knew that every 20 minutes she would be able to sit down somewhere and rest. Her symptoms included widespread pain in all her muscles as well as general fatigue. "I was always too tired to exercise. Besides, I hurt all over and couldn't imagine doing anything I didn't really have to do," said Annette. "Then I began seeing a new doctor and he suggested I try exercising in the pool at a local health club. It's only been a few weeks, but already I notice an improvement in my energy level. My goal is to be able to see an art exhibit and be able to walk around for at least 30 or 40 minutes without thinking about myself. I just want to enjoy the show!"

Disability in old age usually means poor quality of life, substantial medical costs, and dependence on formal and informal caregivers as well as the increased risk of declining health. Regaining previously lost abilities also has a strong, positive psychologic effect on both patients and families that cannot be underestimated.

---

note:

For complete information about exercises geared toward mature adults visit the following site: ***www.nia.hih.gov/exercisebook/chapter4_strength.htm***

For a free copy of the illustrated exercise guide write:
NIA Information Center
P.O. Box 8057
Gaithersburg, MD 20898-8087
Request Publication No. NIH 99-4258

The International Council on Active Aging links to sites for mature consumers interested in health and fitness. **http://www.icaa.cc/Index.asp**

3307 Trutch Street,
Vancouver BC
V6L 2T3
Phone: 604-734-4466
Toll Free: 866-335-9777

Research shows that making even modest efforts to increase physical activity can help maintain and often partly restore proficiency in the weakened functions of endurance, strength, balance and flexibility.

Some people neglect exercising because they are under the impression that to do so one would have to join a health club or invest in expensive equipment. However, that is not the case. All anyone needs are well-fitting, sturdy shoes and loose, comfortable clothing. Recent studies by the National Institutes of Health show significant improvements in health and stress reduction by persons who simply take regular 30-minute walks. Thousands of older adults have eagerly adopted mall-walking as their exercise of choice. They find that the enclosed area is climate-controlled, secure and an abundant resource for making new friends.

Tai chi

Countless numbers of older adults have enthusiastically embraced the practice of tai chi, an ancient form of meditative exercise that originated in China. Tai chi enhances body awareness and those who participate regularly in this practice increase their flexibility while strengthening the muscles used for posture and balance. There is a compelling safety factor associated with tai chi. Students are trained to be aware of their physical limitations as they focus on maintaining stable footing while perfecting balance ability. With practice, there is a rewarding improvement in balance and overall well-being. Tai chi is an ideal complement to traditional programs of walking and resistance training.

Dementia and exercise

The progression of dementia not only affects intellectual abilities but steadily erodes one's motor skills. The damage is done primarily to the complex mechanism in the brain that helps to keep the body upright and which governs movement, balance and walking. As a result, all persons with dementia are at a high risk for falls so it is especially important that they avail themselves of any additional protective benefits exercise has to offer. There are, of course, ample other reasons that dementia patients often fall and some of the better known are:

- Side effects of a prescribed medication. (see table 7.2 p.118)
- Interactions of the multiple drugs being used to treat coexisting illnesses.
- Decline in the ability of the body to excrete drugs because of the weakening function of the aging heart, liver and kidneys.
- Visual impairment.
- Wandering tendencies.
- Environmental hazards.

Exercise cannot cure dementia but it can go a long way to support older adults in their struggle with the steady advance of symptoms. A regular walking program, for example, will improve bowel and bladder function as well as release tension. Furthermore, as the leg and hip muscles are strengthened, there is less likelihood of falls. Those who do exercise regularly report fewer feelings of isolation and a heightened sense of being more in control of day to day living, a feeling they find to be extremely rewarding.

Clinicians note that their dementia patients who exercise appear to be less agitated and more emotionally stable. Caregivers say they see a reduction in pacing, improved sleep at night and a longer retention of their loved one's motor skills.

Exercise for caregivers

Asking caregivers if they exercise will often provoke a terse reply about other, more pressing demands on their time. Having the responsibility for a dementia patient not only means that the caregiver may be sleep deprived but there is frequently the possibility of having elevated blood pressure reactions to stress, a factor strongly associated with heart disease. Furthermore, studies show that the emotional strain accompanying family caregiving is an independent mortality risk for older caregivers. Still, everyone understands that exercise is a fundamental way of remaining physically fit. What is less well known, however, is the fact that regular exercise tailored to the needs of caregivers can help to lower stress-induced blood pressure levels and improve sleep quality.

In the November, 2001 issue of the Journal of Gerontology the results of a landmark study done by a group of Stanford University scientists were highly significant. The researchers found that caregivers who exercised for 30 to 40 minute sessions four times a week were more effectively controlling their stress, reducing blood pressure and improving their energy levels than the control groups who did not exercise. The basis of their success seemed to be the fact that the exercise programs were tailored to the caregivers' preferences. For example, some caregivers who participated were not able to leave the person for whom they were caring, so an individualized indoor program was developed for them. The program was successful primarily because it met the caregivers' needs.

Dr. Sidney M. Stahl, Chief of Behavioral Medicine within the US National Institute of Aging's Behavioral and Social Research Program said, "studies show that family caregiving accompanied by emotional strain is an independent risk factor for mortality among older adults. The study gives us some evidence that a self-directed exercise program can reduce stress reactions and perhaps improve the health of caregivers."

Drugs, dizziness and accident prevention

Although everyone tries to avoid accidents some of the physical changes brought about by aging make the opportunities for mishaps more probable. Auditory and visual changes combined with muscle weakness, impaired coordination and slower reflexes conspire to increase an older adult's chances of falling. Furthermore, most elderly are following complex medical regimens because they have several chronic illnesses. It is widely known, for example, that persons over 65 take between 9 and 13 medications on a daily basis and more than 75 percent of this group are estimated to medicate themselves with unknown numbers of over-the-counter (OTC) medications. When all this information is put in perspective, it is easy to see how the side effects of drugs can heighten an older adult's chance of falling.

note:

Questions to ask a doctor and pharmacist about all medications:

What are the common side effects?
What should be done if a dose is missed?
Are there any foods, drugs, or activities that should be avoided while taking the medication?

Classification:	Generic name:
Antihypertensives	
1. ACE inhibitors:	lisinopril enalapril captopril
2. Vasodilators:	hydralazine isosorbide dinitrate
3. Calcium channel blocker	nifedipine
4. Beta blockers:	metoprolol
Anxiolytics (antianxiety drugs)	alprazolam oxazepam lorazepam
Antidepressants	sertraline citalopram paroxitine venlafaxine
Antiparkinsonian	levodopa carbidopa+levodopa
Cardiac drugs	diltiazem verapamil
Steroids	prednisone dexamethasone
Diuretics (water pills)	furosemide bumetanide hydrochlorthiazide

Table 7.2 Some drugs that can cause dizziness.

Table 7.2 is an abbreviated list of some of the more commonly prescribed drugs that older adults take to control their many chronic illnesses. Nevertheless, self medication with OTC drugs is a commonplace and risky practice that needs to be corrected. As an example, there is the dangerous potential for drowsiness and confusion lurking in most cold and cough medicines, antihistamines, nonsteroidal anti-inflammatory drugs (NSAIDS) and in any drug that contains alcohol (ex. popular OTC cough mixtures).

How can dizziness or feeling faint be avoided? First, a general warning: anyone who feels dizzy or faint should not drive or attempt any activity that requires sustained, careful attention such as using sharp implements, cooking, ironing, or using stairs. Other precautions necessary for older adults to practice are:

- Drinking sufficient fluids in order to avoid dehydration.
- Being active enough to assure good circulation.
- Not smoking and limiting or omitting alcohol.
- Moving slowly when getting out of bed or rising from a prolonged period of being seated.
- Acting prudently when the weather is hot and humid by taking frequent breaks, drinking plenty of fluids and dressing appropriately.

---

note:

More commonsense practices:

Use a night light in the bedroom and bathroom.

Before standing up first thing in the morning, or if getting out of bed during the night, sit on the edge of the bed for a few moments.

Remember, all medications should be reviewed at each physician's visit. It is the best time to ask about adjusting a drug's dosage or replacing it with another medication if an impaired elder experiences drowsiness, confusion or dizziness.

Taking nonprescription drugs responsibly

An ever-expanding selection of nonprescription, OTC drugs has allowed the public to take a more active role in personal health care. The OTC medicines offer many opportunities to take care of the less serious aches and illnesses that are very likely to appear with age. But, by self medicating, people also assume the responsibility to become better informed of the consequences.

The subject of elders' use of nonprescription drugs is critically important to address because so many seniors are strongly influenced by persuasive media advertising. OTC drugs are not benign substances, yet most older adults are dangerously unaware of the effects these substances can have on the body.

The US Food and Drug Administration, Center for Drug Evaluation and Research warns that the very same instructions physicians give their patients for prescription drug use also apply to nonprescription drugs:

- Read the label, know the name of the product.
- Learn what the active ingredients are.
- Understand the purpose of the drug. Know what category it is: antihistamine? cough suppressant? laxative?
- Understand fully the purpose of taking the drug. What symptom or disease will it treat or prevent?
- Ask a pharmacist or physician how the OTC drug will interact with any prescription medications taken.

Consumers can order a free pamphlet, Think It Through: A Guide to Managing the Benefits and Risks of Medicines, from the Center for Drug Evaluation and Research by going online at:

http://www.fda.gov/cder/consumerinfo/think.htm

For those without Internet access, the same information can be obtained by calling:

1-888-INFO-FDA (1-888-463-6332)

or writing to:

US Food and Drug Administration
5600 Fishers Lane
Rockville MD 20857-0001

Another resource is The National Patient Safety Foundation which provides online materials, suggestions and links that can help improve patient safety in the delivery of health care.
http://www.npsf.org/ or info@npsf.org

National Patient Safety Foundation®
515 N. State Street
Chicago, IL 60610
312/464-4848
312/464-4154 (fax)

Certain changes in an aging body can increase the risk of unwanted and possibly harmful drug interactions. The natural, age-induced alteration in body composition, i.e., weight, shape and muscle tone, affects the way drugs are distributed and used. As aging progresses, it is customary for fat distribution to increase and muscles to become smaller and weaker. It is far easier at this time than it ever was before for older adults, particularly sedentary older adults, to gain weight. Women are especially prone to gain weight since they are "fattier" to begin with. (Men have proportionately more muscle than fat.) Although exercise increases the possibility of successful weight control because it burns more calories and tends to suppress appetite, it is not a substitution for decreasing the caloric intake of those who are overweight.

Weight gain is always undesirable because it places added stress on heart, lungs, and the weight bearing joints e.g., knees, hips, ankles, and feet. Sedentary, overweight elders will find it more difficult to climb stairs, get in and out of a car, get out of a chair and simply walk comfortably and safely. Furthermore, weakened muscles cannot protect joints or help to provide the necessary strength and balance essential for use in daily activities. Fortunately, however, the situation can be reversed at almost any age. Impaired elders have many choices of physical activities for improving muscular strength, endurance and flexibility and a suitable program can be developed for anyone.

Osteoporosis

As mentioned earlier, regular exercise maximizes the ability of elderly people to maintain much of their independence and for the longest possible time. It also allows for the rebuilding and repairing of bones so important in the prevention of osteoporosis, commonly called the "brittle bone disease" and so extensive in elderly women. Osteoporosis is insidious because the victims are generally unaware of any symptoms until they sustain a fracture. This extremely common bone disease progresses subtly over the years as bone tissue steadily deteriorates. The resulting bone fragility leads to the increased chance of a fracture and osteoporosis is responsible for more than 1.5 million fractures annually. In spite of the fact that osteoporosis is more widespread in elderly women, it is not unknown in older men. Older adults need to ask their physicians about calcium and vitamin D supplements to improve bone health and vitamin B12 to optimize nerve function.

---

note:
One out of every two white women will experience an osteoporotic fracture at some point in her lifetime.

The most common fractures are those affecting the hip, spine and wrist. Although some fractures may be followed by full recovery, the alternative is chronic pain, disability and even death. The hip fracture is the most serious, with a 20 percent mortality rate within one year.

Moreover, large numbers of hip fracture patients require long term care and only one third ever fully gain their former level of independence.

As patients struggle with pain, physical limitations, depression and lifestyle changes, the anxiety and inevitable dependency associated with these fractures places extraordinarily severe stress on family relationships.

The role of nutrition

There is a world of difference between food that satisfies hunger and food that really nourishes the body. In order to be termed "well nourished" people need to eat and drink enough of the substances required by the body for energy and good health. The basis of good nutrition for older adults is adequate hydration and the consumption of protein, fats, and carbohydrates along with vitamins and minerals in recommended amounts.

Caregivers know that they should be as attentive to their own nutritional needs as they are to the requirements of the one receiving care. Unfortunately, it is very easy to develop poor eating habits because of some of the common situations that can interfere with health maintenance.

loneliness

Social isolation and depression can cause anyone to lose interest in preparing or eating regular meals. Dementia caregivers are also tired after shopping, preparing and serving meals, and at times, feeding their patients. Nevertheless, some adjustments to the meal schedule can help. Smaller, more frequent meals that consist of familiar favorites can appeal to both caregiver and patient. Since eating is a largely social pastime, conversation should be encouraged. However, if that becomes impractical, listening to the radio or music on a stereo can make mealtimes more enjoyable.

lack of motivation (or skill) to cook

Elderly men in particular who never had to cook until their wives became disabled, may snack irregularly or rely on take-out food for their meals. Both habits easily lead to the consumption of calorie-ridden foods made up of excess fats and sugar and with an insufficient supply of vitamins, minerals and fiber.

Help is available in the US under The Older Americans Act which provides nutrition and other services for older people who are in social and economic need. Home delivered meals and congregate dining are the main nutrition programs. Meals On Wheels delivers dinners to homebound individuals and arrangements can be made through a local area agency on aging. Congregate meals programs are widely available in churches, schools, local senior centers and community centers.

Some communities also provide a grocery shopping service for homebound elders. In this program the recipient pays for the groceries and there is usually a service fee.

There are many inexpensive cookbooks available that explain the basic steps for meal preparation and some are published in large print. The US Department of Agriculture sponsors Cooperative Extension Programs in most state universities. These programs offer basic cooking and nutrition workshops and more information can be obtained through a local area agency on aging or by calling the Eldercare Locator Hotline at 1-800-677-1116.

note:

The Eldercare Locator Hotline is active Monday through Friday, 9:00AM - 8:00PM eastern time; voicemail after hours. Caller should be prepared with the address and zip code of the elder in need of services.

Useful websites for nutrition and food safety are found at:
www.fda.gov
http://vm.cfsan.fda.gov
www.foodsafety.gov
http://vm.cfsan.fda.gov/~dms/seniorsd.html

A Consumer Information Catalog offering free or very low cost publications on a wide variety of subjects including food, meal preparation, and healthy eating can be ordered at:
www.pueblo.gsa.gov or by calling 1-888-8 PUEBLO

A choice of international geriatric and social protection sites can be located at the following links:

http://www.healthyeating.net/he_6-02.htm
http://www.von.ca/english/News/meals.htm
http://www.northamptonshire.gov.uk/council/information/guide/mealsonwheels.asp
http://www.nswmealsonwheels.org.au/national.htm
http://europa.eu.int/comm/employment_social/missoc2001/index_en.htm

The Food and Drug Administration Hotline and the USDA Meat and Poultry Hotline can answer food safety questions as well as other questions about food issues consumers may have at:

1-888-SAFEFOOD and 1-800-535-4555

The US Department of Agriculture maintains a food and nutrition information center at 1-301-504-5719.

financial constraints

Many older adults live on a fixed income and lack of money often leads to stinting on certain nutrient-rich food purchases such as meat, fish, fresh fruits and vegetables. (Money problems are also reasons older adults delay dental and medical visits that might correct barriers to good nutrition.) Food stamps, the coupons that consumers redeem for food in stores, are an underutilized source of nutrition assistance for low-income elderly. Although food stamps can increase their purchasing power, there are several reasons many eligible retirees, including veterans, neglect to participate:

- They are unaware that the program exists.
- They feel that there is a social stigma to being a welfare recipient.
- They are misinformed about the program and assume they are ineligible if they are homeowners or do not have dependent children.
- They perceive that the application process is cumbersome, not worth the effort for what seems to be low benefits.

The Commodity Supplemental Food program sponsored locally in the US provides food for low-income elderly. Food packages consisting of canned fruits and vegetables, meats, fish, peanut butter, cereal, grains and dairy products are labeled to indicate the product's nutritional content. Specific information is available from the local senior centers.

---

note:
Community service organizations are in the White Pages of the local telephone directory.

Similar programs are provided abroad and information can be found at:
http://europa.eu.int/comm/employment_social/missoc2001/index_en.htm

The website **www.benefitscheckup.org** is a quick way to determine eligibility for a wide range of benefits. The Nation Council on the Aging sponsors this site to help people find programs that can pay for some of the costs of prescription drugs, health care, utilities, and other essential services. The results are confidential.

There is also a useful fact sheet available online to determine income eligibility for food stamps for the elderly and disabled and this can be checked at:

www.fns.usda.gov/fsp/regulations/elderly&disabled.htm

People in need of more information or who wish to apply for food stamps should contact a local food stamp office. This is listed under "Human Resources," "Social Services," or "Food Stamps" in the state or local government pages of the telephone directory. Each state has a food stamp hotline for information on the program. To find that number, call the Food Stamp hotline at: 1-800-221-5689. Persons with Internet access can visit the web site at **http://www.fns.usda.gov/fsp.**

International inquiries can be made at:
http://www.elderweb.com/orginfo.php?OrgID=1454

Other Barriers to good nutrition

Many elderly individuals do not eat foods that are important for good health because of chewing difficulties and certain gastrointestinal disturbances. Missing teeth and ill-fitting dentures often mean that fresh fruits and vegetables, valuable sources of vitamins, minerals and fiber, are left out of the daily diet. When dairy products are avoided because the older adult believes they cause gas or constipation, some important sources of calcium and protein are omitted. In addition to the decrease of taste and smell that normally occurs with aging is the fact that medications can also impair these senses.

medical factors

While a busy caregiver may be tempted to take shortcuts and rely heavily on "fast foods", they are assuming unnecessary risks if the basic steps of good nutrition are omitted. The Food Guide Pyramid (Figure 7.1) was developed by the US Department of Agriculture (USDA) as a visual display that is easy for consumers to read. It is important to balance the food consumed with physical activity. The Food Guide Pyramid displays general categories of foods to eat based on nutritional guidelines.

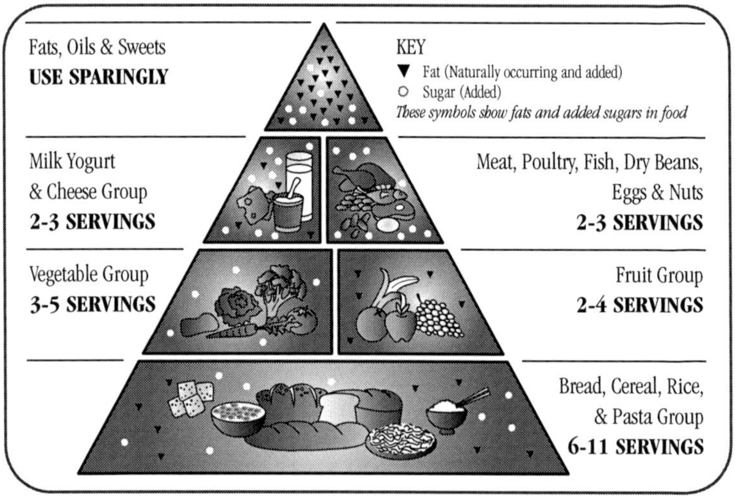

Figure 7.1 The Food Guide Pyramid.
Source: U. S. Department of Agriculture, Department of Health and Human Services.

A diet that is moderate in salt and sodium to help reduce the risk of high blood pressure would feature the following characteristics:

- Food choices that are limited in sugars. A diet with an abundance of sugar has too many calories and too few nutrients for most people and can contribute to tooth decay.
- Liberal selection of grain products, vegetables, and fruits which provide necessary vitamins, minerals, fiber, and complex carbohydrates that can help to lower fat intake.
- Foods that are low in fat, saturated fat, and cholesterol to reduce the risk of heart attack, and certain types of cancer. A low fat diet also helps one to achieve and maintain a healthy weight.

It should be everyone's goal to maintain or improve weight in order to reduce the chances of developing high blood pressure, heart disease, stroke, certain cancers, and diabetes.

Older adults also need to limit alcohol consumption since alcohol supplies calories but no nutrients. More important, alcohol interacts poorly with medications and is also the root of many physical and mental health problems.

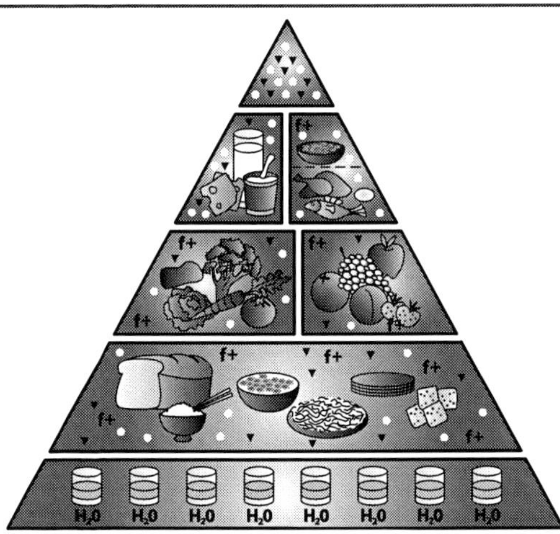

Figure 7.2 Modified Food Guide Pyramid for Adults over Seventy Years.
Source: Tufts University; U. S. Department of Agriculture, Department of Health and Human Services.

Researchers at Tufts University investigated the dietary needs of the population of elderly adults over seventy and modified the food guide pyramid. The modifications as shown in Figure 7.2, allow for the reduced energy needs of an elderly person, yet it accurately reflects the nutritional requirements of today's elderly with the implication that since fewer calories are needed, the nutritional value of each calorie is particularly important. That principle is the basis for the key differences in the adjusted food pyramid:

- The modified pyramid indicates nutrient-dense choices in all food categories.
- It stresses the importance of fiber and adequate hydration.
- It suggests the possible need for dietary supplements - namely, calcium and vitamin D to improve bone health and vitamin B12 to optimize nerve function.

Managing problem behavior

As the symptoms characterizing dementia advance, caregivers often encounter troubling behaviors at mealtime. Once-fastidious loved ones can become messy and even hide food in inappropriate places. Others will refuse food, or else demand to eat shortly after the meal is over claiming that they never were served! No matter how disturbing as this type of conduct is, there are ways of managing it. As an example, if using a knife and fork is no longer practical, supply mostly finger foods, cut meat into small manageable pieces or offer whatever is to be eaten with a spoon. Some additional helpful suggestions are:

- Toilet the person before the meal and minimize distractions. For some, television is a distraction but familiar music playing softly is generally relaxing.
- Cover clothing with a large cloth or sturdy paper napkin.
- Offer food that is easily chewed and safely swallowed.
- Limit the number of dishes offered. Some individuals are more confused with a tray filled with several different servings, but will manage well if offered one food item at a time over the course of the meal.

Brain impairment can also affect the ability to swallow. Be sure to allow the person plenty of time to eat and modify the texture of the foods to accommodate poor chewing and swallowing behaviors. A soft diet is safer and often more acceptable for the person with advanced dementia than a regular diet that requires very careful eating patterns. Make use of thickening agents that can be added to liquids to reduce choking hazards. Calorie-laden, vitamin-rich supplements are widely available and should be incorporated into the diet between meals for those patients whose intake is not adequate.

Caregivers are continually challenged by their loved one's abrupt departures from acceptable, traditional behavior. Uncontrollable outbursts stem from being confronted by a situation that is overwhelming at that time. As hard as it is for families to accept, the patient is not being obstinate or willful. As the brain becomes more impaired the ability to evaluate situations or adapt behavior appropriately diminishes. Patients in the later stages of dementia are unable to control their reactions and shouting, crying or aggressive conduct are common. An unimpaired person has more socially acceptable ways of managing pressure, frustration or fatigue. As caregivers, family members and friends become attuned to what circumstances can provoke tantrums, they can gradually reduce these occurrences and diffuse potentially explosive situations.

CHAPTER 8

Caregiving

According to reliable estimates published by the European Parliament, by the year 2020, fully twenty five percent of the EU population will be over 65 years of age. The number of people over 80, the group at highest risk for physical and mental disabilities, will increase even more. Taken in this context demographers forecast a 300 percent increase in the numbers of people over 80 between 1960 and 2020.

Nearly 25 percent of Americans 65 and older are disabled or dependent on some form of long term care. More than 8 million people over age 70 need help to manage their daily lives. They are not so severely impaired that they need to be institutionalized, but they do need some kind of assistance so that they can function at home. Currently, more than one third of elderly people who live in the community have unmet daily activities needs. The American Academy of Actuaries projects that by the year 2040, the population of severely disabled elderly will increase by 90 percent. By that is meant that they will need help with their personal care e.g., bathing, dressing, toileting as well as the more complex tasks that most of us we do automatically such as cooking, banking, and traveling about. If the services of family caregivers had to be replaced with paid services, the cost would be nearly $200 billion per year.

Who are the people who are saving the government this enormous sum? They are a severely stressed population known as the sandwich generation who are the adult children of frail elders and who have children of their own and who provide nearly half of the care. Elderly spouses, who are usually struggling with their own health problems, furnish about 25 percent. Predictably, most of the caregivers report that their many (and often unfamiliar) responsibilities cause them both physical and emotional strain.

Nevertheless, caregivers seldom plan adequately for the future. They do not anticipate needs or plan early enough how they will provide care for elderly parents and they also do not plan for changes in caregiving requirements. The well known maxim to "take one day at a time" is a standard coping strategy, but that only works when the situation is stable or changes slowly.

As family caregivers assume more and more of their responsibilities, most have said that they wish they had been better prepared to provide care. As they take on their roles, most have expressed regret that they did so lacking information about the resources that exist, how to get help for their loved ones and themselves, and how they could improve their own quality of life. However, no one who is thrust into the caregiving role is ever fully prepared. Consequently, many care recipients have expressed concern about the health and well-being of their caregivers.

When dementia is irreversible highly specialized care is needed and few families are equipped to manage both their lives and the lives of their afflicted loved ones without this alternative. Looking after a person with dementia is all consuming and totally unlike other types of caregiving. As a group, dementia caregivers report more problems at work, more physical and mental health issues, more inter-family conflicts and less time available to spend with other family members than caregivers in nondementia situations.

These caregivers are continuously faced with intensely challenging situations that require specific managing techniques. The areas that seem to generate the most stress are primarily behavior management, safety precautions and legal considerations:

behavior management

The disruptive behaviors of dementia that characteristically develop as the illness advances are the most frequent reasons for institutionalization. Family caregivers become increasingly frustrated, exhausted, and even frightened by their their loved one's hallucinations, sleep disturbances, agitation and aggression. As a result, they may regard nursing home placement as the only solution. This is not to suggest that nursing home placement is ever a sign of failure. Rather, it is another phase of the illness continuum. Living with someone who has a dementing illness commonly leads a caregiver to determine that there is more to be gained by all concerned if the responsibility is relinquished to skilled health care professionals for the following reasons:

- It is the patient's best interest in terms of health and safety.
- The primary caregiver can no longer manage caregiving with work and family responsibilities.
- The primary caregiver's personal problems with age and health preclude continuing to look after the patient in a home setting.

Inappropriate behavior and memory problems make it extremely difficult to guide and protect an impaired individual at home. Sometimes the challenges are more than the caregiver can manage. However, there are some practical strategies that caregivers can try in order to keep their loved one at home as long as possible.

Table 8.1 illustrates common behavior problems in people who have dementia, how they are manifested, and suggested solutions.

safety precautions

Families' safety measures can range from improving lighting and reducing the hot water temperature to lowering thresholds between rooms and installing outdoor ramps. However, these decisions are usually made promptly because they are so obviously practical. The more disturbing issues may involve an individual's independence. As examples, who decides when the patient should stop driving, working, or living alone? These difficult, perplexing questions should be

problem:	**presentation:**	**caregiver response:**
hallucinations	Seeing, hearing, smelling, tasting,or feeling something no one else perceives.	If the hallucination is not causing anxiety, do nothing. If the patient is upset, try to distract or redirect his attention. Inform the doctor as they may be drug-related. Continued hallucinations can be managed with specific medication.
agitation, aggression	Pacing, resisting care, crying, trying to hit caregiver.	Assess situations that seems to trigger the behavior. Simplify tasks. Ex. if the person refuses to shower in the morning, try the evening. Schedule a shower every other day. Limit choices. Reduce the stimulation of sounds, avoid crowds.
sleep disturbances	day/night reversal	Orient the person to day and night. Encourage some form of exercise daily. Have a clock prominently displayed. Open drapes so sun or or darkness is readily visible. Limit caffeine consumption and have quiet evening activities. Determine if sleeplessness is pain related. Toilet regularly.

Table 8.1 behavioral problems and solutions.

addressed by the person's physician or a medical practitioner familiar with the family's situation. As a rule when high risk behavior is identified, it must be curbed immediately and consequently, some activities must stop abruptly. Nonetheless, the primary physician weighs the caregiver's assessment of the patient's behavior before any fundamental lifestyle activities are altered.

legal considerations

Financial management and the creation of an advance directive, a document that sets up durable power of attorney and living will, require the specialized attention of professionals.

These issues are addressed in Chapter 1., p.13. However, problems can arise when an individual is a resident of a nursing home and has any mental and/or physical impairments. A recent study determined that such persons might not have their preferences honored. In order to avoid this, families and nursing staff need to work together and communicate clearly and often in order to respect and ensure the residents' preferences.

Help and support for the caregiver

Despite such changes in family life as the soaring numbers of women working and the increased likelihood of geographic separation, family involvement has been unflagging. There is widespread research documenting the fact that caregivers devote about 20 hours weekly looking after older persons and much more time when someone has multiple disabilities. Shouldering these burdens is extremely stressful both physically and emotionally.

In the US, The National Family Caregiver Support Program, launched in 2000, is a federal plan of action to help support families to sustain their efforts to looking after their ailing elderly relatives. The program has five components:

1. The provision of information to caregivers about available services.
2. Outreach to caregivers so that they are able to access such services.
3. Individual counseling, organization of support groups, provision of caregiver training to help families make decisions and solve problems generated by their responsibilities.
4. Respite care to provide temporary relief from caregiving responsibilities.
5. Supplemental long term care services for a limited period of time to complement the care families provide for their loved ones.

A local Area Agency on Aging (or US Department of Elder Affirs) is one of the first resources a caregiver should contact when help is needed. These offices are listed in the city or county government sections of the telephone directory.

The following website gives a fuller explanation of both the aging network and National Family Caregiver Support Program: **http://www.aoa.gov/carenetwork/default.htm**

The toll-free Eldercare Locator service which operates Monday through Friday, 9:00 a.m. to 8:00 p.m., Eastern time, can be reached at 1-800-677-1116. This resource has been helping elders and their caregivers find local aid agencies for information and referral since 1991.

Some helpful resources that apply to caregivers internationally can be found at:

http://www.eurohealth.ie/remind/index.htm
http://www.alzheimer.ca/english/care/caregivers-intro.htm
http://www.planetamber.com/scripts/go/29220

note:
For other international resources, please see appendix 1.

The average caregiving situation is that of a responsible family member totally absorbed in the care of a loved one to the degree that personal needs are often neglected. Typically, this person is a women who not only has a job and family of her own but who is also taking care of an elderly parent. The extra help extended ranges from shopping, cleaning and personal care to home repairs, transportation and medication and financial management.

Not surprisingly, these demands become overpowering which then compromises the caregiver's physical and emotional health as well as that of the frail dependent elder. When the care involves someone with a dementing disorder, the pressures are magnified in frequency, duration, and intensity. Caregivers need to understand they are not expected to shoulder all these responsibilities by themselves and that they are entitled to explore potential resources in the following ways:

- Ask for help with a situation that is harder to manage than anyone could have anticipated. Discuss strategies with family members. Neighbors and friends of the elderly person can become involved if they are informed about the circumstances.

- Recognize when it is time to make use of community services, (see Area Agency on Aging and Eldercare Locator, p.6) then do it. Maintaining ties with elderly parents who live far away is especially difficult. However, using the services of a geriatric care manager is often a satisfactory solution.

  For a more complete explanation log on to: **http://www.caremanager.org/**

  The official headquarters is at:

  National Association of Professional Geriatric Care Managers
  1604 N. Country Club Road
  Tucson, AZ 85716-3102
  520-881-8008
  520-325-7925 FAX

- Investigate the Employees Assistance Programs in the workplace. Many companies offer help in the form of flexible schedules, referrals, counseling and seminars on caregiving.

As indicated in the December 15, 1999 issue of the Journal of the American Medical Association, caregiving responsibilities exert a major influence on the health of the caregiver. The never ending daily stresses can cause depression, anxiety, and a variety of physical ailments. Moreover, in the case of an elderly caregiver burdened with the responsibility of a disabled spouse, the mental and physical strain related to caring can be life threatening.

Most caregiving stress can be traced to three broad issues:

1. Behaviors of the affected individual.
2. Lack of family support.
3. Not using respite care.

behaviors

Caregivers can learn to understand that certain behaviors, primarily, repeating the same questions over and over, wandering, and pacing are caused by a brain disease that progresses slowly and is often unpredictable. The caregivers' stress escalates as the behavior increases in frequency and intensity.

(Please refer to table 8.1 and appendix 3.)

family support

A family meeting led by a physician or trained counselor can be a positive approach toward mobilizing their group support. An objective, third party who meets with the family in neutral territory (an office) can appraise the situation while diffusing emotional responses. This is an appropriate time for suggesting practical, effective management, choices and plans that are in the dementia patient's best interests.

respite care

The concept of respite care may not be fully understood by caregivers because it has several meanings. It can be the use of adult day care twice a week, a neighbor who spends an hour or two with the older adult so that the caregiver can keep a dental appointment, or a nursing home admission for a full week so a caregiver can spend some time away from the elder.

Respite programs may be underutilized. However, there is mounting evidence to suggest that the incidence of care-related stress and depression is significantly lower when family caregivers regularly avail themselves of some type of respite care.

Maintaining well-being, managing stress

Most of us are fully aware that living a healthy lifestyle requires getting enough sleep, eating a balanced diet, exercising, and enjoying favorite outside interests. Caregivers are no exception. However, the day to day concerns of the health and safety of their elderly charge can override the power to be objective about personal well-being. If the pressure and stress of weighty responsibilities are unrelieved there will be serious threats to the quality of life.

Caregivers owe it to themselves and their families to take measures that will preserve their physical and mental health. Some tips include:

- Maintaining optimal nutrition.
- Getting enough sleep.
- Making exercise a part of daily life.
- Setting aside some time for socializing.
- Accepting support from family, friends, and professionals.
- Pursuing the services available in the community.

Adult children find it upsetting to watch their parents age while battling the many physical and mental health issues that contribute to frailty and decline. The later years place increasing strains on family relationships and accordingly, caregivers need to continually reevaluate their positions as they search for workable solutions to problems. They are hardworking people who live with uncertainty and are always contending with stress. Coping is easier said than done because the strong emotional ties can subtly cloud objectivity. Nevertheless, strategies that deal with anger, stress, and frustration can help diffuse volatile situations and maintain the strength of family bonds. Some commonsense measures to use are:

- Understand that feelings of frustration, stress, and anger are normal.
- Restrict alcohol intake.
- Join a caregiver support group.
- Call a hotline.
- Walk away from the stressful situation even if it is just to another room for a few minutes.
- Utilize respite care. This can range from informal help from family, friends, or church groups to adult day care and short term nursing home admission. There are several states that subsidize respite care for qualifying individuals, e.g., frail elder, Alzheimer's disease, low-income or Medicaid eligible, as well as some community-based free respite centers. Contact a local Area Agency on aging (in the telephone directory under state or county government listings) or call the Eldercare Locator number 1-800-677-1116.

---

note:

Through the AoA's new National Family Caregiver Support Program, hundreds of thousands of families across the United States are receiving community-based support, training and assistance in caring for a family member who is disabled or chronically ill.

There are caregivers who learn to unburden themselves by writing their thoughts and feelings in a journal. They find that this practice seems to provide an emotional release by helping them view troubling situations in a different light and with more objectivity.

Stress has an important function because it fuels our motivation and can keep us goal oriented. Yet, individual responses to stress differ and, as expected, some people manage their daily life pressures better than others. When writing identifies a stress trigger the caregiver can then focus on developing an effective strategy to manage it.

Caregivers claim that the benefits of keeping a journal are rewarding because:

- It fosters the development of emotional detatchment.
- It helps to keep the severity of incidents in perspective.
- It advances the setting of realistic goals.
- It reinforces successful strategies.

Some caregivers have also learned to practice relaxation techniques by focusing on meditation and deep breathing exercises that calm and relax the mind and body. By learning to recognize which stressors are environmental, interpersonal, or in the case of the employed caregiver, job related, techniques can be often developed to eliminate the source or reduce the impact of the stress.

Families have found that they are able to reduce some of the chaos and confusion in their lives not only by simplifying tasks, but by identifying problem areas in the home and making a few simple, practical changes. Often it may be something as easy as closing a door because this will limit the dementia patient's access to other rooms. When clutter and unnecessary furniture are removed, safety is increased, anxiety is lessened, and caregiving becomes easier. A less distracting environment also helps to keep the patient happier and more independent.

Stress is always intensifed when coping is unsuccessful. Nevertheless, developing tactics that either reduce the pressures of caregiving or increase the carer's level of tolerance is not only satisfying but more important, empowering.

Spirituality and caregiving

Many people regard religion and spirituality as being one and the same. However, there is a marked distinction: religion implies rules, holy rituals, and pious teachings while spirituality is open to a much broader yet no less important interpretation. Spirituality refers to one's personal search for the meaning of life. A report from the 1971 White House Conference on Aging asserted that "all persons are spiritual, even if they have no use for religious institutions and practice no personal pieties." It is understood that all those who practice a religion are not necessarily spiritual and that many deeply spiritual persons may not be affiliated with a specific religion.

Anyone who works with older adults sees that there are large numbers of frail elderly who find comfort and meaning in their lives through their relationships with family and friends. Others may use religious rituals and teachings to support and reaffirm their own spirituality.

The last few years has seen a burgeoning emphasis on the importance of having a spiritual outlook reported in mainstream medical journals as well as in the popular press. A well known current example is author David Snowdon's powerful book about his unique Alzheimer's disease research investigations called Aging With Grace. Dr. Snowdon combined the high-tech scrutiny of the brain with a heartwarming story of the aging nuns being studied. When commenting on the nuns' spirituality he says that "profound faith, like a positive outlook, buffers the sorrows and tragedies that all of us experience. There is evidence available from other sources suggesting that prayer and contemplation have a positive influence on long-term health and may even speed the healing process." The capability of religion and spirituality to affect physical and mental health has gained international interest and recognition.

Caregivers naturally center their attention on the dementia patient's physical health. Among their chief concerns are:

- Providing good nutrition.
- Encouraging participation in some form of exercise.
- Helping to conserve the elder's cognitive function.
- Maintaining a safe environment.

This emphasis is certainly appropriate and should be supported. However, there is a spiritual dimension of life that is also vitally significant to all older adults, and the patient with dementia is no exception. Most of today's elderly population have had a religious affiliation at some time in their lives. It does not matter if frailty precludes an active participation in religious services, religion is still an essential component of quality of life.

Spiritual reinforcement helps to reassure an impaired person that their life, however restricted, is still meaningful. Although it may be difficult to determine exactly what someone with dementia can understand, spiritual practices are usually quite comforting and frequently can allay fears. This, in turn, reduces anxiety and frustration. Nonetheless, some caregivers and clinicians are hesitant when it comes to addressing a patient's spiritual needs. The reasons for this are unclear, but it is possible they feel that spirituality is a private matter or at least that it should be confined to a place of worship. Then too, there may have been family conflicts about religion and personal spirituality in the past. There is also the likelihood of mixed feelings about individual spiritual values or their absence.

Whatever the reason, both patient and caregiver benefit significantly when spiritual needs are met. Whether through traditional religious prayer or by means of meditation and conversation, if the practice is used in a non-judgmental accepting manner both parties gain in the development of one of the strongest available coping mechansims.

Intercessory prayer

No mention of meeting spiritual needs would be complete without referring to intercessory prayer, e.g., the practice of having one person pray for another in order to promote the healing process.

There have been many studies suggesting support for the premise that prayer helps to enhance the healing process in patients. Furthermore, prayer, meditation, deep breathing exercises or relaxation techniques are all effective methods for cultivating spirituality and offering patients and their caregivers some peace and comfort.

The driving dilemma

The majority of older adults care passionately about maintaining their independence and all of them dread declining cognitive function as well as any other threat to their autonomy and the quality of their lives. When the diagnosis of dementing illness is made, patients and their families are overwhelmed by having to face the review of all aspects of daily living ranging from the management of medications and finances to matters of dress and hygiene. Driving is another daily activity that most people take for granted, and being compelled to stop can be devastating. Resentment builds, guilt grows and all persons involved suffer the consequences.

Driving is the standard way of getting about in today's mobile society. It is not only a widely recognized symbol of independence and control but more important, when dementia is the diagnosis, it is an activity that demands immediate review since driving while impaired can be life threatening. Any discussion about losing driving privileges is guaranteed to be one of the most highly charged, emotional issues facing both patients with cognitive deficits and their caregivers. Nevertheless, it is absolutely imperative that any elderly drivers who are hazardous behind the wheel be prevented from driving.

Dementing disorders present unique problems when compared to other types of disability. As examples, drivers who have visual deficits or mobility problems can often manage quite well with the appropriate adaptive devices. Despite the fact that dementia is a serious issue, there may be a period of time in the very early stages of the illness when the person can drive safely with caregivers monitoring the situation in the following ways:

- Confining driving to familiar destinations (ex. nearby churches, markets, hairdressers).
- Limiting the distance to drive.
- Driving only during daylight hours.
- Using alternate transportation in bad weather.

Early diagnosis and improved medication add to the increased possibility of more minimally affected elderly drivers. Unsurprisingly, most of the information about dementia counsels against driving, yet precisely how or when to stop is generally left up to patients and their caregivers because there are no enforceable standards applicable to these frail elderly drivers.

Most elderly drivers stop driving of their own accord when they are ready. However, people with dementia have little if any insight into their own driving capability or the accidents their impairment can cause. The subtle, unpredictable course of a dementing illness renders the affected individual unable to assess their own capacity for driving safely with any measure of reliability. This places the responsibility squarely on the shoulders of either an adult child or elderly spouse, whichever is the caregiver. At some point that person must decide between their loved one's independence and self esteem and the public safety. The following points may help family members to clarify their reasoning:

- Even if your loved one is driving in a familiar area, unpredictable circumstances are bound to occur.
- The rate of cognitive decline cannot be precisely determined.
- There is no way to determine at what point the older adult passes from being a safe driver to being dangerous.

Decreasing driving opportunities, suggesting alternatives

Early in the illness caregivers can enlist the support of other family members, friends and neighbors to drive the older adult to occasional appointments and religious or social events. Certain items and commodities can be delivered, namely, medications, and meals. Many hairdressers, podiatrists, and other health care personnel will make house calls. Virtually all banking services are automated. As the need for driving is reduced and alternatives are used more frequently, the actual relinquishing of the car can be done with dignity intact.

Caregivers who begin a discussion by insisting that the driver turn over the car keys forthwith, will almost certainly meet stoney resistance or perhaps explosive anger. However, if concerns are phrased as questions rather than as demands the chance of a confrontation will be diminished. The following suggestions can introduce the subject of hazardous driving and its consequences, while paving the way for acceptable alternatives:

- Ask how the elderly driver feels about the stress of traffic, dealing with less experienced and more careless drivers, and the increased likelihood of facing emergencies i.e., a child darting into the road.
- Determine if the driver really understands his prescriptions and any potential side effects such as as a slowing of one's reaction time and drowsiness.

- Prepare a comparison of the annual cost of insurance, fuel, and vehicle maintenance to that of public transportation and taxi fares.
- Find out through a social agency if there is a community van service.
- Research specialized transportation services through local taxi companies. Many offer a senior discount.

These suggestions are appropriate only if the individual is in the early stages of the dementing illness and can still understand the consequences of driving while impaired. As the disorder advances, caregivers must step up the efforts toward alternative transportation.

Although they cannot reliably predict driving competence, (an on-road assessment is the most valid means of such a judgment) clinicians are in a good position to diffuse a family crisis by make a firm recommendation that the patient discontinue driving because of physical or mental limitations. This approach allows an individual to surrender driving privileges gracefully and with dignity intact.

Occasionally, however, situations arise that are not so successfully resolved:

Harry, 87, flatly refused to stop driving after being diagnosed with a dementing illness. He ignored the entreaties of his son who lived in another state and the advice of his physician. Despite numerous fender-benders, tickets for illegal parking, and soaring increases in his insurance he was undeterred. Eventually he had a serious accident while in his own driveway. He hit an elderly neighbor who was about to get into the car with him and the extent of the woman's injuries caused her lengthy hospitalization.

When his son was notified, he immediately drove to his father's home, confiscated the car keysand disabled the car. He then went to the department of motor vehicles (DMV) with the police report. Harry's physician followed up with a letter of recommendation to stop driving because of physical and mental circumstances. The DMV proceeded to issue a notice to Harry requireing him to retake the driving exam.

As it turned out, the DMV appointment was never kept. Harry's dementia advanced rapidly and the son soon had to place him in a nursing home. The injured woman is also in a nursing home and her family has retained an attorney.

In Harry's case, it is likely that the cascade of events could not have been avoided. Nevertheless, older adults and their families need to acknowledge their responsibilities and anticipate adverse events and create some type of plan for the protection of the elderly driver, pedestrians and other motorists.

Maintaining/encouraging independence

Throughout the life span there are always threats and barriers to one's independence. All of us value our independence because it is a quality that has such a strong association with identity or 'personhood'. Today's elderly have developed a variety of uaeful coping skills as they accumulated years of experiences managing disappointments, changes, and losses over the years. Any review of such cataclysmic events as the Great Depression, World War 2, and the sweeping international upheavals that followed, only emphasizes the extraordinary resilience of the current elderly population. Nonetheless, old age is also a time when elders are most sorely tested trying to maintain the independence they achieved after the labors of a lifetime. Mindful of this, families of dementia patients firmly support their loved one's efforts to function at the highest level for as long as they possibly can.

With early intervention and appropriate care many infirm elderly can extend their years of independence. An important and often overlooked first step to individualized care and attention is the validation of the individual's dignity and quality of life by health care professionals. Respectful terms of address and good listening skills on the parts of clinicians and their associates can set the tone for fuller, more meaningful communication.

Caregivers are advised to watch for alterations in their loved one's behavior. Examples of changes that demand prompt professional attention are:

- Impairment in carrying out activities of daily life, e.g., bathing, dressing, toileting, food preparation, medication management.
- Lack of personal hygiene, an kempt appearance.
- Neglected personal responsibilities (unopened mail, unpaid bills, accumulations of trash, missed appointments).
- Social withdrawal.
- Decline in mental abilities, e.g., confusion, personality changes, memory lapses, poor judgment.

Even in the face of declining skills and abilities, the impaired patient should be persuaded to do as much for himself as he possibly can. It does not matter that tasks are incomplete or done poorly, it is the attempt that is important because it is that effort which builds self-esteem and reinforces a sense of fulfillment.

An important goal of dementia care is supporting the affected person's struggle to maintain those characteristics that define their individuality. Caregivers are continually being challenged to strike a safe balance between maintaining safety and encouraging the dementia patient to remain independent. There is a risk that the complexities of diagnosis and treatment, symptom management, caregiver circumstances, and financial factors can, at times, overshadow efforts to keep the identity of the dementia patient intact.

Future directions

In 1980 the total number of people in the world with dementia was 11 million. In the year 2000 the figure rose to 18 million and the projection for 2025 could reach 34 million. This global demographic transformation will have deep-felt consequences on multiple levels: social, economic, cultural and political. Some of the areas of research include:

- Fuller descriptions of normal aging.
- Improved diagnoses for cases of dementia.
- Research combining imaging, psychological testing, and pathological aspects of cognitive decline.
- Development of 'smart' drugs that target the stages of dementia and an Alzheimer's vaccine.
- Examination of the ethical issues that raise serious social questions that need to be addressed, e.g., genetic testing, insurance and legal concerns, issues of disclosure, end-of-life care

At the 8th International Conference on Alzheimer's and Related Disorders that was held in Stockholm, July, 2002, it was noted that attendance since the inaugural conference in 1988 had grown more than 12 fold – from 300 scientists to nearly 3700 from 78 countres. In just the last two years research presentations have nearly doubled. The presentations reflected a striking increase in the investigation of potential Alzheimer risk factors, including elevated cholesterol and blood pressure, nutrition, tobacco and alcohol use, exercise, and body weight.

In 1988 there were no presentations about drug treatment. In contrast, 2002 featured a wealth of studies describing fresh insights about drugs in current clinical trials, new drugs under development and basic cellular and molecular processes affected by drug therapy.

The conference focused international attention on dramatic evidence of the growing worldwide prominence and success of dementia research.

There is also increasing attention being given to the development and implementation of sorely needed social and economic assistance for family caregivers.

A Canadian study looked at tax relief and pension programs in Canada and other countries highlighting the need to evaluate the benefits of tax credits to caregivers. In the US, the Lifespan Respite Care Act has been passed by the House of Representatives and is presently before the Senate. This bill would amend the Public Health Service Act to establish a program to assist family caregivers to access affordable and high-quality respite care as well as for other purposes. The Act would allow nearly $730 million in grants over five years to organizations that initiate or expand respite care programs. Examples are that state and local agencies, as well as some nonprofit organizations, would have funds to recruit and train respite care workers and family caregivers. These organizations and agencies would also encourage and assess further research of services that could relieve some of the responsibilities borne by family caregivers.

A brief summary of global challenges includes:

- The well known changing sociodemographics of the older population - the aging baby boomers who are also the "sandwich generation".
- Projected changes in active life expectancy and concentration of disability; more needs for care but for shorter periods of time at advanced ages.
- The ability of families, which will be smaller and older, to care for the oldest-old and severely disabled elders.
- The increased ethnic diversity of populations stressing the need for culturally sensitive services.

Families are heavily burdened by the intensity of the caregiving experience. The sobering figures of the projected increases in the elderly population in the coming decades, must capture the attention of health care professionals and help to form the goals of those who develop policies, benefits and services for all caregivers.

APPENDIX 1

Quick Fixes for Managing Problem Behaviors

Behavior:	Strategy:
Anger/agitation	Limit or omit caffeine from the diet. Reduce noise, eliminate clutter. Restrict number of people in the room. Keep furniture in the same place. Use gentle touch, hand massage, soothing music. Speak in a reassuring voice. Limit choices. (ex. "here is your sweater" not "which sweater do you want to wear" Divert the individual with a snack. Take the individual to the bathroom.
Incontinence	Establish a toileting schedule. Begin with guiding the individual to the bathroom every 2 hours. Identify the bathroom with a large picture on the door. Monitor fluid intake, e.g., limit evening fluids, avoid drinks that can have a diuretic effect (coffee, tea, beer, carbonated beverages). Use clothing that is easy to remove ex. pants with elastic waistbands and washable. Use commercial incontinence products. Ask a urologist about the feasibility of treatment.
Wandering	Consider electronic devices made specifically to monitor this type of behavior. Secure doors with locks that are unfamiliar to the individual. Install sensors that signal when a door is opened. Have an ID bracelet made for the person and maintain a current photo. Inform neighbors of tendency to wander and leave a contact phone number with them. Plan on regular exercise to reduce restlessness and tension.

Behavior:	Strategy:
Pacing	Encourage the individual to move and exercise. Reassure her if she feels lost and remind her that she is in the right place. Give her something to do: stacking papers, folding laundry, winding yarn.
Paranoia	Help the person look for a missing object. Use redirection. Try reassuring non-verbally with gentle touch, or a hug while making eye contact. Ask physician about patient's medications and the possibility of side effects.
Repetitive speech, questions or movements	Try reassurance or distraction. Place large signs in obvious places "I will phone you at 4PM" "Tom is coming here at 7PM." Large pictures also help, ex. picture of toilet on bathroom door. Confirm with physician that the individual is not in pain or experiencing side effects of a drug.

SPECIAL CONCERNS

Bathing

Skip a day if bathing becomes a problem. Dementia patients can lose the ability to distinguish hot water from cold which causes anxiety. Try a sponge bath. There are also pleasant commercial products marketed for this purpose.

Change the time of day for bathing by varying the time to meet the patient's needs. Always supervise showers and baths. Remove door lock for safety.

Clothing

Limit choices. Lay out clothing one item at a time to encourage independence and reduce indecision and anxiety. Choose loose, comfortable attractive clothing that feels pleasing to the touch. Immediately remove soiled clothing to avoid having the patient insist on wearing it.

Eating

Dementia patients lose the ability to remember when they have eaten. Conceal food when it is not meal time. Serve pre-cut foods when the individual has difficulty managing utensils. If the person insists he has not had his meal, try distraction with another activity.

Agitation at bedtime

Keep the home well lit until bedtime. Allow for some type of exercise during the day. Use soft, soothing music and hand/arm/back massage while getting the patient into nightclothes. Have a night light in the bedroom and quick access to a commode at the bedside. If the problem increases, consider hiring a night aide and ask the physician if some medication at bedtime would be helpful.

WHAT NOT TO DO

Do not attempt to restrain the individual during outbursts.

Do not use confrontation during or after a troubling incident.

Avoid discussing any plans until just before the event takes place.

Avoid negative sentences, loud angry tones of voice.

Do not insist on discussing events or people the individual no longer remembers.

APPENDIX 2

Sample of a Geriatric Depression Scale

Questions:	Mark Y/N	Answer
1. Are you basically satisfied with your life?	Yes / No	**No**
2. Have you dropped many of your activities or interests?	Yes / No	**Yes**
3. Do you feel that your life is empty?	Yes / No	**Yes**
4. Do you often get bored?	Yes / No	**Yes**
5. Are you in good spirits most of the time?	Yes / No	**No**
6. Are you afraid that something bad is going to happen to you?	Yes / No	**Yes**
7. Do you feel happy most of the time?	Yes / No	**No**
8. Do you feel helpless?	Yes / No	**Yes**
9. Do you prefer to stay at home, rather than go out and do things?	Yes / No	**Yes**
10. Do you feel that you have more problems with memory than most?	Yes / No	**Yes**
11. Do you think it is wonderful to be alive now?	Yes / No	**No**
12. Do you feel pretty worthless the way you are now?	Yes / No	**Yes**
13. Do you feel full of energy?	Yes / No	**No**
14. Do you feel that your situation is hopeless?	Yes / No	**Yes**
15. Do you think that most people are better off than you are?	Yes / No	**Yes**
Total Score		

Scoring: assign one point for each of the test answers.

A score of 0 - 5 is normal. A score above 5 suggests depression and a more thorough clinical investigation should be undertaken.

Yesavage JA Brink TL Rose TL et al. Development and validation of a geriatric depression screening scale: a preliminary report. J. Psychiatr. Res. 1983; 17:37-49.

Source: National Institute of Aging, National Institutes of Health Womens Health and Aging Study, 1995
http://www.nia.nih.gov/health/pubs/whasbook/chap8/tab83.pdf

APPENDIX 3

Additional international sites:

Alzheimer's Disease International lists national associations at:
http://www.alz.co.uk/help/associations.html

Alzheimer Europe This site exists in English, French, Greek, Italian and German
http://www.alzheimer-europe.org/

Alzheimer's Association Australia The Association represents, at the national level, the interests of its federation of members in each State and Territory on all matters relating to dementia and carer issues. Its mission is to improve the quality of life for people with dementia.

Alzheimer's Association Australia: http://www.alzheimers.org.au/
Alzheimer's Association New South Wales: http://www.alznsw.asn.au/

Alzheimer Society of Canada - Société Alzheimer du Canada - A national non-profit organization to help Canadians affected by Alzheimer Disease. The latest information on Alzheimer care, research and Society programs. Support and forums for caregivers and physicians. **http://www.alzheimer.ca/** Sites offer a language choice of French or English.

Canadian Mental Health Association
2160 Yonge, 3rd floor - 3e étage
Toronto, ON M4S 2Z3
Tel./Tél.: (416) 484-7750
Fax: (416) 484-4617
Email: national@cmha.ca

a detailed listing of other CMHA Provincial Offices & Regions, please visit CMHA National's web site at **http://www.cmha.ca/english/info_centre/locations.htm**

http://www.alz.uk/help click on "Find the Alzheimer's association in your country". This shows the international site that lists countries of the world alphaabetically with names addresses, phone numbers fax, email addresses and websites

http://www.alznebraska.org/docs/Library.html
All-inclusive library of references and guides for Alzheimer's disease and related dementing disorders: videos, children's books, slides etc.

APPENDIX 4

Example of a mental status examination: The Short Portable Mental Status Questionnaire (SPMSQ)

Questions:	Response	Incorrect Responses
1. What are the date, month, and year?		
2. What is the day of the week?		
3. What is the name of this place?		
4. What is your phone number?		
5. How old are you?		
6. When were you born?		
7. Who is the current president?		
8. Who was the president before him?		
9. What was your mother's maiden name?		
10. Can you count backward from 20 by 3's?		

SCORING: *

0-2 errors: normal mental functioning

3-4 errors: mild cognitive impairment

5-7 errors: moderate cognitive impairment

8 or more errors: severe cognitive impairment

*One more error is allowed in the scoring if a patient has had a grade school education or less.
*One less error is allowed if the patient has had education beyond the high school level.

Source: Pfeiffer, E. (1975). A short portable mental status questionnaire for the assessment of organic brain deficit in elderly patients. Journal of American Geriatrics Society. 23, 433-41.

Compiled by the Lincoln/Greater Nebraska Chapter of the Alzheimer's Association, 1999. Used with permission.

BIBLIOGRAPHY

Agostini JV, Leo-Summers LS, Inouye SK. Cognitive and other adverse effects of diphenhydramine use in hospitalized older patients.Arch Intern Med. 2001 Sep 24;161(17):2091-7.

Aguero-Torres, Fratiglioni L, Guo Z, Viitanen M, von Strauss E, Winblad B. Dementia is the major cause of functional dependence in the elderly - 3-year follow-up data from a population-based study. Am J Pub Health 1998; 88:1452-1456.

Aisen PS. Evaluation of selective COX-2 inhibitors for the treatment of Alzheimer's disease. J Pain Symptom Manage. 2002 Apr;23(4 Suppl):S35-40.

Ala TA, Hughes LF, Kyrouac et al The Mini-Mental State exam may help in the differentiation of dementia with Lewy bodies and Alzheimer's disease. Int J Geriatr Psychiatry. 2002 Jun;17(6):503-9.

Alagiakrishnan, A. Vascular dementia. Oct. 18, 2001 eMedicine

Aldridge D. Spirituality, healing and medicine.Br J Gen Pract. 1991 Oct;41(351):425-7

Alexopoulos GS, Meyers BS, Young RC, Kakuma T, Silbersweig D, Charlson M. Clinically defined vascular depression. Am J Psychiatry. 1997;154:562-565.

Alexopoulos G Bruce M Hull J Sirey J Kakuma T Clinical Determinants of Suicidal Ideation and Behavior in Geriatric Depression. Arch Gen Psych 1999 Nov;56: 1048

Allard CG. Advances in the treatment of Alzheimer's disease: benefits of dual cholinesterase inhibition. Eur Neurol. 2002;47(1):64-70.

Allison M, Keller C. Physical activity in the elderly: benefits and intervention strategies. Nurse Pract. 1997 Aug;22(8):53-4, 56, 58

Ancill J, Sheldon LJ, Nielsen RJ. Depression versus dementia. Can J Psychiatry. 1993 Mar;38(2):155-6.

Anderson DN. Treating depression in old age: the reasons to be positive. Age Ageing. 2001 Jan;30(1):13-7.

Andrieu S, Reynish E, Nourhashemi F, et al Predictive factors of acute hospitalization in 134 patients with Alzheimer's disease: a one year prospective study. Int J Geriatr Psychiatry 2002 May;17(5):422-6

Appels A. Depression and coronary heart disease: observations and questions.J Psychosom Res. 1997 Nov;43(5):443-52.

Arai Y, Zarit SH, Sugiura M, Washio M. Patterns of outcome of caregiving for the impaired elderly: a longitudinal study in rural Japan. Aging Ment Health. 2002 Feb;6(1):39-46.

Arendash GW, Gordon MN, Diamond DM, et al Behavioral assessment of Alzheimer's transgenic mice following long-term Abeta vaccination: task specificity and correlations between Abeta deposition and spatial memory. DNA Cell Biol. 2001 Nov;20(11):737-44.

Bai DL, Tang XC, He XC Huperzine A: Potential Therapeutic Agent for Alzheimer's Disease. Curr Med Chem 2000 Mar;7(3):355-74

Baartels SJ, Levine K, Horn S, Sharkey P: Treatment of depression in older primary care patients in health maintenance organizations. Int J Psychiatry Med 1997;27:215-232

Bas A Veld I Ruitenberg A et al Nonsteroidal Antiinflammatory Drugs and the Risk of Alzheimer's Disease Volume 345:1515-1521 November 22, 2001 Number 21 NEJM

Bayyreuther K, Masters CL. Molecular biology and prevention of Alzheimer's disease -- esperiments and strategies. Program and abstracts of the 17th World Congress of Neurology; June 17-22, 2001; London, UK. J Neurol Sci. 2001;187(suppl 1): S116.

Beeson R, Horton-Deutsch S, Farran C, Neundorfer M. oneliness and depression in caregivers of persons with Alzheimer's disease or related disorders. Issues Ment Health Nurs. 2000 Dec;21(8):779-806.

Benbow SM. Management of depression in the elderly. Br J Hosp Med. 1992 Dec 2-1993 Jan 5;48(11):726-31

Bird MJ, Parslow RA Potential for community programs to prevent depression in older people. Med J Aust. 2002 Oct 7;177(7 Suppl):S107-10.

Blakeman TM, Comino EJ, Zwar NA, Harris MF. Evaluating the introduction of the enhanced primary care 75+ annual health assessments. Aust Fam Physician 2001; 30: 1004-1009.

Bland RC. Psychiatry and the burden of mental illness. Can J Psychiatry 1998;43:801-10.

Blazer DG. Depression in the elderly. Myths and misconceptions. Psychiatr Clin North Am. 1997 Mar;20(1):111-9.

Bliwise DL. Sleep apnea, APOE4 and Alzheimer's disease 20 years and counting? J Psychosom Res. 2002 Jul;53(1):539-46.

Bonner LT, Peskind ER. Pharmacologic treatments of dementia. Med Clin North Am. 2000 May; 86(3):657-74.

Bourgeois, M., Schulz, R., & Burgio, L. Interventions for caregivers of patients with Alzheimer's disease: A review and analysis of content, process, and outcomes. International Journal on Aging and Human Development 1996; 43, 35-92.

Bourke J, Castleden CM, Stephen R, et al. A comparison of clock and pentagon drawing in Alzheimer's disease. Int J Geriatr Psychiatry 1995;10:703_705.

Bowen J, Teri L, Kukull W, et al. Progression to dementia in patients with isolated memory loss. Lancet 1997;349:763_765.

Brink TL, Yesavage JA, Lum O, Heersema P, Adey MB, Rose TL: Screening tests for geriatric depression. Clinical Gerontologist 1: 37-44, 1982.

Brodaty H, Howarth GC, Mant A, Kurle SE. General practice and dementia. A national survey of Australian GPs. Med J Aust 1994; 160: 10-14.

Brodaty J, Draper B, Lie D; Psychogeriatrics and general practice in Australia. Int J Psychiatry Med 1997;27: 205-214

Brodaty H, Griffin D, Hadzi-Pavlovic D. A survey of dementia carers. Doctors' communications, problem behaviours, and institutional care. Aust N Z J Psychiatry 1990; 24: 362-370.

Brown JS, Vittinghoff E, Wyman JF et al . Urinary incontinence: Does it Increase Risk for Falls and Fractures? Journal of the American Geriatric Society 2000; 48, 721-725.

Brown CK Spirituality, healing and medicine. Br J Gen Pract. 1992 Jan;42(354):39.

Bruce D, Paterson A. Barriers to community support for the dementia carer: a qualitative study. Int J Geriatr Psychiatry 2000; 15: 451-457.

Bruce DG, Paley GA, Underwood PJ, Roberts D, Steed D. Communication problems between dementia carers and general practitioners: effect on access to community support services. Med J Aust. 2002 Aug 19;177(4):186-8.

Buchner DM, Cress ME, de Lateur BJ, et al The effect of strength and endurance training on gait, balance, fall risk, and health services use in community-living older adults. J Gerontol A Biol Sci Med Sci. 1997 Jul;52(4):M218-24.

Bullock R. The clinical benefits of rivastigmine may reflect its dual inhibitory mode of action: an hypothesis. Int J Clin Pract. 2002 Apr;56(3):206-14 49-52, 55.

Burgener S, Twigg P. Relationships among caregiver factors and quality of life in care recipients with irreversible dementia. Alzheimer Dis Assoc Disord. 2002 Apr-Jun;16(2):88-102.

Butler RN, Lewis MI Late-life depression: when and how to intervene. Geriatrics 1995 Aug;50(8):44-6,

Canadian Psychiatric Association. Canadian clinical practice guidelines for the treatment of depressive disorders. Can J Psychiatry 2001;46:Supp1

Butler RN, Going overboard with mini-mental exams. Geriatrics. 1989 Feb;44(2)15

Cahn DA, Salmon DP, Butters N, et al. Detection of dementia of the Alzheimer type in a population-based sample: neuropsychological test performance. J Int Neuropsychol Soc 1995;1:252_260.

Carney R Freedland K Jaffe A Depression as a Risk Factor for Coronary Heart Disease Mortality. Commentary. Arch Gen Psych 2001 March; 58 (3)

Carta A Calvani M Bravi D Ni Bhuachalla S. Acetyl-L-carnitine and Alzheimer's disease: Pharmacological beyond the cholinergic sphere. Ann. New York Acad. Sci. 1993 69(5/): 324-326

Castro CM, Wilcox S, O'Sullivan P, Baumann K, King AC. An exercise program for women who are caring for relatives with dementia. Psychosom Med. 2002 May-Jun;64(3):458-68.

Cerrato PL. Alternatives. Complementary therapies--Spirituality and healing. RN. 1998 Feb;61(2):49-50.

Challis D, von Abendorff R, Brown P, Chesterman J, Hughes J. Care management, dementia care and specialist mental health services: an evaluation. Int J Geriatr Psychiatry. 2002 Apr;17(4):315-25.

Chalmers J. Global impact of stroke.Heart Dis. 2000 Mar-Apr;2(2):S13-7.

Chandler JM, Zimmerman SI, Girman CJ, et al Low bone mineral density and risk of fracture in white female nursing home residents. JAMA. 2000 Aug 23-30;284(8):972-7.

Charlton R, Sheahan K, Smith G, Campbell I. Spousal bereavement--implications for health. Fam Pract 2001 Dec;18(6):614-8

Chertkow H, Bergman H, Wolfson C, LeBlanc A, Murtha S, McKelvey R. Natural history and prediction of progression in mild cognitive impairment. Program and abstracts of the 17th World Congress of Neurology; June 17-22, 2001; London, UK. J Neurol Sci. 2001;187(suppl 1): S9.

Chodosh J, Reuben DB, Albert MS, Seeman TE. Predicting cognitive impairment in high-functioning community-dwelling older persons: MacArthur Studies of Successful Aging. J Am Geriatr Soc. 2002 Jun;50(6):1051-60.

Clegg A, Bryant J, Nicholson T, et al Clinical and cost-effectiveness of donepezil, rivastigmine and galantamine for Alzheimer's disease: a rapid and systematic review. Health Technol Assess. 2001;5(1):1-137.

Cohen J. The Global Burden of Disease Study: a useful projection of future global health? J Public Health Med 2000 Dec;22(4):518-24.

Costa PT, Jr., Williams TF. Development of clinical practice guidelines for dementia screening. Neurobiology of Aging 1992;13:S5.

Czaja SJ, Rubert MP. Telecommunications technology as an aid to family caregivers of persons with dementia. Psychosom Med. 2002 May-Jun;64(3):469-76.

Dalton JE, Pederson SL, Blom BE, Holmes NR. Diagnostic errors using the Short Portable Mental Status Questionnaire with a mixed clinical population. J Gerontol. 1987 Sep;42(5):512-4.

Dawson C, Whitfield H. ABC of urology. Urinary incontinence and urinary infection. BMJ. 1996 Apr 13;312(7036):961-4.

Day L, Fildes B, Gordon I, et al Randomized factorial trial of fall prevention among older people living in their own homes. BMJ. 2002;325(7356):128-134

Dello Buono M, Busato R, Mazzetto M, et al. Community care for patients with Alzheimer's disease and non-demented elderly people: Use and satisfaction with services and unmet needs in family caregivers. Int J Geriatr Psychiatry 1999; 14: 915-924.

De Marco RR. The epidemiology of major depression: implications of occurrence, recurrence, and stress in a Canadian community sample. Can J Psychiatry 2000;45:67-74.

Deschamps V, Barberger-Gateau P, Peuchant E, Orgogozo JM Nutritional factors in cerebral aging and dementia: epidemiological arguments for a role of oxidative stress. Neuroepidemiology. 2001 Feb;20(1):7-15.

Drachman DA, Swearer JM. Driving and Alzheimer's disease: the risk of crashes. Neurology 1993; 43: 2448-2456.

Dugue M, Neugroschl J. Anxiety disorders. Helping patients regain stability and calm. Geriatrics. 2002 Aug;57(8):27-31.

Edwards AB, Zarit SH, Stephens MA, Townsend A. Employed family caregivers of cognitively impaired elderly: an examination of role strain and depressive symptoms. Aging Ment Health. 2002 Feb;6(1):55-61.

Eisenberg, L "The World Burden of Mental Illness," APA Symposium, Toronto, Canada, June 1998.

Emre M. Switching cholinesterase inhibitors in patients with Alzheimer's disease. Int J Clin Pract Suppl. 2002 Jun;(127):64-72

Englander F, Hodson TJ, Terregrossa RA. Economic dimensions of slip and fall injuries. J Forensic Sci 1996 Sep;41(5):733-46

Evans WJ. Exercise training guidelines for the elderly. Med Sci Sports Exerc. 1999 Jan;31(1):12-7.

Ewbank, D. Deaths Attributable to Alzheimer's Disease in the United States. American Journal of Public Health (January 1999), v. 89(1), pp. 90-92.

Farlow MR Pharmacokinetic profiles of current therapies for Alzheimer's disease: implications for switching to galantamine. Clin Ther. 2001;23 Suppl A:A13-24.

Farlow MR. Do cholinesterase inhibitors slow progression of Alzheimer's disease? Int J Clin Pract Suppl. 2002 Jun;(127):37-44.

Feeney DM, Tarlow B, Jones RN et al Factors affecting the use of telephone-based intervention for caregivers of people with Alzheimer's disease. Telemedicine, Journal and E-Health: The Official Journal of the American Telemedicine Association 2001 7(3), 139-48

Ferrari E, Casarotti D, Muzzoni B, et al Age-related changes of the adrenal secretory pattern: possible role in pathological brain aging. Brain Res Rev 2001 Nov;37(1-3):294-300

Fiatarone MA, et al. Exercise training and nutritional supplementation for physical frailty in very old people. N Engl JMed 1994;330:1769-1775.

Fichter MM, Meller I, Schroppel H, Steinkirchner R. Dementia and cognitive impairment in the oldest old in the community. Prevalence and comorbidity. Br J Psychiatry. 1995 May;166(5):621-9.

Fink A, Hays RD, Moore AA, Beck JC. Alcohol-related problems in older persons. Determinants consequences, and screening.Arch Intern Med. 1996 Jun 10;156(11):1150-6.

Fisk JD, Rockwood K, Hondas B, et al. Cognitive screening in a population-based sample of community-living elderly: effects of age and education on the construct of cognitive status. Int J Geriatr Psychiatry 1995;10:687_694.

Fitten LJ, Perryman KM, Wilkinson CJ, et al. Alzheimer and vascular dementias and driving. JAMA 1995; 272: 1360-1365.Am Geriatr Soc 1993; 41: 747-53.

Foley DJ, Monjan AA, Masaki KH,et al Associations of symptoms of sleep apnea with cardiovascular disease, cognitive impairment, and mortality among older Japanese-American men. J Am Geriatr Soc. 1999 May;47(5):524-8.

Folstein MF, Folstein SE, McHugh PR. Mini-Mental State. A practical method for grading the cognitive state of patients for the clinician. J Psychiatr Res 1975;12:189_198

Fox GK, Bowden SC, Bashford GM, Smith DS. Alzheimer's disease and driving: prediction and assessment of driving performance. J Am Geriatr Soc 1997; 45: 949-953.

Fox N, Crum WR, Scahill R, Rossor MN. Patterns of tissue loss in degenerative dementia detected with voxel compression mapping of serial MRI. Where does atrophy in Alzheimer's disease start and how does it progress? Program and abstracts of the 17th World Congress of Neurology; June 17-22, 2001; London, UK. J Neurol Sci. 2001;187(suppl 1): S116.

Frade, S The Global Impact of Dementia July, 2001 Signpost Magazine

Fratiglioni L, Launer LJ, Andersen K, et al, for the Neurologic Diseases in the Elderly Research Group. Incidence of dementia and major subtypes in Europe: a collaborative study of population-based cohorts. Neurology. 2000;54(suppl 5):S10-S15.

Frenkel D, Solomon B. Towards Alzheimer's beta-amyloid vaccination. Biologicals. 2001 Sep-Dec;29(3-4):243-7.

Fried LP, Guralnik JM. Disability in older adults - Evidence regarding significance, etiology and risk. J Am Geriatr Soc 1997;45:92-100.

Friedman SM, Williamson JD, Lee BH, et al Increased fall rates in nursing home residents after relocation to a new facility. J Am Geriatr Soc. 1995 Nov;43(11):1237-42.

Gallo J, Rabins PV, Illiffe S: The 'research magnificent' in late life: Psychiatric epidemioloogy and the primary health care of older adults. Int J Psychiatry Med. 1997;27:215-232

Gallo J Ryan S Ford D Attitudes, Knowledge, and Behavior of Family Physicians Regarding Depression in Late Life 1999; May/June Arch Fam Med. (8): 249

Gao S, Hendrie HC, Hall KS, et al. The relationships between age, sex, and the incidence of dementia and Alzheimer's disease. A meta-analysis. Arch Gen Psychiatry 1998;55:809_815. 10.

Gauthier S. Controversies in therapy. Program and abstracts of the 17th World Congress of Neurology; June 17-22, 2001; London, UK. J Neurol Sci. 2001;187(suppl 1): S118.

Gatz M, Svedberg P, Pedersen NL et al Education and the risk of Alzheimer's disease: findings from the study of dementia in Swedish twins. J Gerontol B Psychol Sci Soc Sci. 2001 Sep;56(5):P292-300.

Geldmacher DS. Cost-effective recognition and diagnosis of dementia. Semin Neurol. 2002 Mar;22(1):63-70.

Gelenberg A. Depression is still underrecognized and undertreated. Arch Intern Med. 1999 Aug 9-23;159(15):1657-8.

Gilley DW, Wilson RS, Bennett DA, et al. Cessation of driving and unsafe motor vehicle operation by dementia patients. Arch Intern Med 1991; 151: 941-946.

Golde TE. Inflammation takes on Alzheimer disease.Nat Med. 2002 Sep;8(9):936-8.

Goldenberg B, Chiverton P. Assessing behavior: the Nurse's Mental Status Exam. Geriatr Nurs 1984 Mar-Apr;5(2):94-8

Golomb J, Wisoff J, Miller DC et al Alzheimer's disease comorbidity in normal pressure hydrocephalus: prevalence and shunt response. J Neurol Neurosurg Psychiatry. 2000 Jun;68(6):778-81.

Greenough WT, Cohen NJ, Juraska JM. New neurons in old brains: learning to survive? Nat Neurosci. 1999;2:203-206.

Greubel DL, Stokesberry C, Jelley MJ. Preventing costly falls in long-term care.Nurse Pract. 2002 Mar;27(3):83-5.

Hageman PA, Thomas VS. Gait performance in dementia: the effects of a 6-week resistance training program in an adult day-care setting. Int J Geriatr Psychiatry. 2002 Apr;17(4):329-34.

Hain TC, Fuller L, Weil L, Kotsias J. Effects of T'ai Chi on balance. Arch Otolaryngol Head Neck Surg. 1999 Nov;125(11):1191-5.

Hartman CA, Manos TM, Winter C, Effects of T'ai Chi training on function and quality of life indicators in older adults with osteoarthritis. J Am Geriatr Soc. 2000 Dec;48(12):1553-9.

Hauer K, Rost B, Rutschle K, Exercise training for rehabilitation and secondary prevention of falls in geriatric patients with a history of injurious falls. J Am Geriatr Soc. 2001 Jan;49(1):10-20.

Hawkins KA, Cooper ME. Limitations of cognitive status exams: a case-based discussion. Psychiatry. 1996 Winter;59(4):382-8.

Hebblewhite J, Finucane P. Aged Care Assessment Teams in Australia: a general practice perspective. Aust J Ageing 1995; 14: 27-30.

Helmuth L. NSAIDS for prevention? Protecting the brain while killing pain? Science. 2002 Aug 23;297(5585):1262-3.

Helmuth L. New therapies. New Alzheimer's treatments that may ease the mind. Science. 2002 Aug 23;297(5585):1260-2.

Henschke PJ. Infections in the elderly. Med J Aust 1993 Jun 21;158(12):830-4

Heun R, Papassofirotoulos A, Jennssen F. The validity of psycho- metric instruments for detection of dementia in the elderly general population. Int J Geriatr Psychiatry 1998;13:368_38

Hofman A, Ott A, Breteler MMB, Bots ML et al Atherosclerosis, apolipoprotein E and the prevalence of dementia and Alzheimer's disease in a population-based study: the Rotterdam Study. Lancet 1997;349:151-154.

Hogan DB, Ebly EM, Fung TS. Disease, disability, and age in cognitively intact seniors - Results from the Canadian Study of Health and Aging. J Gerontol (Med Sci) 1999;54A:M77- M82.

Hooker K, Bowman SR, Coehlo DP et al Behavioral change in persons with dementia: relationships with mental and physical health of caregivers. J Gerontol B Psychol Sci Soc Sci. 2002 Sep;57(5):P453-60.

Hoozemans JJ, Bruckner MK, Rozemuller AJ, et al. Cyclin D1 and cyclin E are co-localized with cyclo-oxygenase 2 (COX-2) in pyramidal neurons in Alzheimer disease temporal cortex. J Neuropathol Exp Neurol. 2002 Aug;61(8):678-88.

Hull M, Lieb K, Fiebich BL. Nonsteroidal drugs and Alzheimer's disease. N Engl J Med. 2002 Apr 11;346(15):1171-3.

Hunt L, Morris JC, Edwards D, Wilson BS. Driving performance in persons with mild senile dementia of the Alzheimer type. J Am Geriatr Soc 1993; 41: 747-53.

Iddon JL, Pickard JD, Cross JJ. et al Specific patterns of cognitive impairment in patients with idiopathic normal pressure hydrocephalus and Alzheimer's disease: a pilot study. J Neurol Neurosurg Psychiatry 1999 Dec;67(6):723-32

Jain, K. K. (2000). "Evaluation of memantine for neuroprotection in dementia." Expert OpinInvestig Drugs 9(6): 1397-406

Jeste, DV, Finkel SI. Psychosis in Alzheimer's disease: Diagnostic criteria for a distinct syndrome (guest editorial) Am J Geriatr Psych 2000; 8:29-34

Johansson K, Bogdanovic H, Kalimo H, et al. Alzheimer's disease and apolipo- protein E e 4 allele in older drivers who died in automobile accidents. Lancet 1997; 349: 1143-1144.

Jones A. Managed care strategy for mental health services. Br J Nurs. 1997 May 22-Jun 11;6(10):564-8.]

Jorm, A; Jolley, D. The Incidence of Dementia: A Meta-Analysis. Neurology (September 1998), v. 51(3), pp. 728-33

Journal of Financial Service Professionals, January 2001. Some Observations About the Senior Citizens' Freedom to Work Act of 2000.

Juva K, Sulkava R, Erkinjuntti T, et al. Usefulness of the Clinical Dementia Rating scale in screening for dementia. Int Psychogeriatr 1995;7:17_24

Kaplan MS, Adamek ME, Martin JL. Confidence of primary care physicians in assessing the suicidality of geriatric patiet Int J Geriatr Psychiatry 2001 Jul;16(7):728-34

Katz I Coyne J The Public Health Model for Mental Health Care for the Elderly 2000 June 7; Vol. 283 No. 21,

Khandelwal SK. Depressive disorders in old age. J Indian Med Assoc. 2001 Jan;99(1):39, 42-4.

Kivipelto M, Helkala E-L, Laakso MP "Apolipoprotein E &egr;4 Allele, Elevated Midlife Total Cholesterol Level, and High Midlife Systolic Blood Pressure Are Independent Risk Factors for Late-Life Alzheimer Disease." An Int Med 2002 Aug 6; (137):149-155.

Knopman DS, DeKosky ST, Cummings JL. et al. Practice parameter: diagnosis of dementia (an evidence-based review). Report of the Quality Standards Subcommittee of the American Academy of Neurology. Neurology. 2001;56:1143-1153.

Kokmen E, Smith GE, Petersen RC, et al. The short test of mental status: correlations with standardized psychometric testing. Arch Neurol 1991;48:725_728

Kornhuber, J., M. Weller, et al. (1994). "Amantadine and memantine are NMDA receptor antagonists with neuroprotective properties." J Neural Transm Suppl 43: 91-104

Krebs DE, Jette AM, Assmann SF. Moderate exercise improves gait stability in disabled elders. Arch Phys Med Rehabil. 1998 Dec;79(12):1489-95.

Kukull WA, Bowen JD Dementia epidemiology. Med Clin North Am. 2002 May;86(3):573-90.

Kurz AF. What is vascular dementia?Int J Clin Pract Suppl. 2001 May;(120):5-8.

Lasser RA, Dukoff R, Levy J, Levin R, Lehtimaki T, Seubert P, Sunderland T. Apolipoprotein E epsilon 4 allele in association with global cognitive performance and CSF markers in Alzheimer's disease. Int J Geriatr Psychiatry. 1998 Nov;13(11):767-74.

Lam R W, Chronic schizophrenia and idiopathic Parkinson's disease. Can J Psychiatry 1993 Mar;38(2):75-77.

Lamb HM, Goa KL. Rivastigmine. A pharmacoeconomic review of its use in Alzheimer's disease. Pharmacoeconomics. 2001;19(3):303-18.

Lebowitz, BD, Pearson, JL, Schneider, Ls et al Diagnosis and treatment of depression in late life. JAMA 1997; 278:1186-1190.

Landes AM, Sperry SD, Strauss ME, Geldmacher DS. Apathy in Alzheimer's disease. J Am Geriatr Soc. 2001 Dec;49(12):1700-7.

Lasser RA, Dukoff R, Levy J, et al Apolipoprotein E epsilon 4 allele in association with global cognitive performance and CSF markers in Alzheimer's disease. Int J Geriatr Psychiatry. 1998 Nov;13(11):767-74

Laurin D Verreault R Lindsay J et al Physical Activity and Risk of Cognitive Impairment and Dementia in Elderly Persons Arch Neurol. 2001;March 58:498-504

Lema MJ. Emerging options with coxib therapy. Cleve Clin J Med. 2002;69 Suppl 1:SI76-84.

Leveille SG, et al. Preventing disability and managing chronic illness in frail older adults - A randomized trial of a community-based partnership with primary care. J Am Geriatr Soc 1998;46:1191-1198.

Leveille SG, Guralnik JM, Ferrucci L, Langlois JA. Aging successfully until death in old age - Opportunities for increasing active life expectancy. Am J Epidemiol 1999;149:654-664.

Levy R. Age-associated cognitive decline. Int Psychoger 1994;6:63_ 68.

Li F, Harmer P, McAuley E, An evaluation of the effects of Tai Chi exercise on physical function among older persons: a randomized contolled trial. Ann Behav Med. 2001 Spring;23(2):139-46.

Lindsay J, Laurin D, Verreault R, et al Risk factors for Alzheimer's disease: a prospective analysis from the Canadian Study of Health and Aging. Am J Epidemiol. 2002 Sep 1;156(5):445-53.

Lipski PS, Driving and dementia: a cause for concern. Med J Aust 1997; 167: 453-454.

Llácer A, Zunzunegui M, Gutierrez-Cuadram P et al Correlates of wellbeing of spousal and children carers of disabled people over 65 in Spain The European Journal of Public Health Volume 12, Issue 1, March 2002: pp. 3-9

Lobo A, Launer LJ, Fratiglioni L, et al, for the Neurologic Diseases in the Elderly Research Group. Prevalence of dementia and major subtypes in Europe: a collaborative study of population-based cohorts. Neurology. 2000;54(suppl 5):S4-S9.

Low LF, Brodaty H, Draper B. A study of premorbid personality and behavioural and psychological symptoms of dementia in nursing home residents. Int J Geriatr Psychiatry. 2002 Aug;17(8):779-83.

Luchsinger JA, Tang MX, Shea S, Mayeux R. Caloric intake and the risk of Alzheimer disease. Arc Neurol. 2002 Aug;59(8):1258-63.

Lyons, K., & Zarit, S. (1999). Formal and informal support: The great divide. Int J Geriatr Psychiatry, 14, 183-196

McCaddon A, Hudson P, Ellis D, Hill D, Lloyd A. Effect of supplementation with folic-acid on relation between plasma homocysteine, folate, and vitamin B12.Lancet. 2002 Jul 13;360(9327):173.

McCusker J, Cole M, Abrahamowicz M, Environmental risk factors for delirium in hospitalized older people. J Am Geriatr Soc. 2001 Oct;49(10):1327-34.

McMurdo ME, Millar AM, Daly F. A randomized controlled trial of fall prevention strategies in old peoples' homes. Gerontology. 2000 Mar-Apr;46(2):83-7.

Mace N, Facets of dementia. Using mental status tests. J Gerontol Nurs. 1987 Jun;13(6):33

Maia L, de Mendonca A. Does caffeine intake protect from Alzheimer's disease? Eur J Neurol. 2002 Jul;9(4):377-82.

Manning RT The serial sevens test. Arch Intern Med 1982 Jun;142(6):1192

Martikainen P, Valkonen T. Mortality after the death of a spouse: rates and causes of death in a large Finnish cohort Am J Public Health 1996 Aug;86(8 Pt 1):1087-93

Matthews DA, Marlowe SM, MacNutt FS. Effects of intercessory prayer on patients with rheumatoid arthritis. South Med J. 2000 Dec;93(12):1177-86.

Mayberg HS, Liotti M, Brannan SK, et al. Reciprocal limbic-cortical function and negative mood: converging PET findings in depression and normal sadness. Am J Psychiatry. 1999;156:675-682.

Mazzeo RS, Tanaka H. Exercise prescription for the elderly: current recommendations. Sports Med. 2001;31(11):809-18.

Meek, P; McKeithan, K; Schumock, G. Economic Considerations in Alzheimer's Disease. Pharmacotherapy (March 1998), v. 2(pt. 2), pp. 68-73 & 79-82

Mehta KM, Yaffe K, Covinsky KE. Cognitive impairment, depressive symptoms, and functional decline in older people. J Am Geriatr Soc. 2002 Jun;50(6):1045-50.

Messier SP, Royer TD, Craven TE, Long-term exercise and its effect on balance in older, osteoarthritic adults: results from the Fitness, Arthritis, and Seniors Trial (FAST). J Am Geriatr Soc. 2000 Feb;48(2):131-133

Meuleman JR. Association of diphenhydramine use with adverse effects in hospitalized older patients: possible confounders. Arch Intern Med. 2002 Mar 25;162(6):720-1.

Mickley JR, Carson V, Soeken KL. Religion and adult mental health: state of the science in nursing. Issues Ment Health Nurs. 1995 Jul-Aug;16(4):345-60.

Mittelman M, Ferris S, Steinberg G, et al. An intervention that delays institutionalization of Alzheimer's disease patients: treatment of spouse-caregivers. Gerontologist 1993; 33: 730-740.

Mittelman MS Ferris SH Shulman E Steinberg G Levin B, A family intervention to delay nursing home placement of patients with Alzheimer's disease. Journal of the American Medical Association, 1996 276(21): 1725-1731.

Mizuno E, Hosak T, Ogihara R, Higano H, Mano Y. Effectiveness of a stress management program for family caregivers of the elderly at home. J Med Dent Sci. 1999 Dec;46(4):145-53.

Monteiro IM, Boksay I, Auer SR et al Reliability of routine clinical instruments for the assessment of Alzheimer's disease administered by telelphone. J Geri Psychiatry Neur 1998 Sspring; 11(1): 18-24

Morris JC. The Clinical Dementia Rating (CDR): current version and scoring rules. Neurology 1993;43:2412_2414.

Mounier N, Andre M, Lepage E. Nonsteroidal drugs and Alzheimer's disease. N Engl J Med. 2002 Apr 11;346(15):1171-3.

Moyle W, Edwards H, Clinton M. Living with loss: dementia and the family caregiver. Aust J Adv Nurs. 2002 Mar-May;19(3):25-31.

Murray CJL, Lopez AD. The Global Burden of Disease: A Comprehensive Assessment of Mortality and Disability From Diseases, Injuries, and Risk Factors in 1990 and Projected to 2020. Cambridge, Mass: Harvard University Press; 1996.

Murray CJLm Lopez AD, Progress and directions in refining the global burden of disease approach: a response to Williams. Health Economics. 2000 9:69-82

Navarro V, Gasto C, Lomena F, Mateos JJ, Marcos T, Portella MJ. Normalization of frontal cerebral perfusion in remitted elderly major depression: a 12-month follow-up SPECT study. Neuroimage. 2002 Jul;16(3 Pt 1):781-7.

Nurmi I, Luthje P. Incidence and costs of falls and fall injuries among elderly in institutional care. Scand J Prim Health Care. 2002 Jun;20(2):118-22.

O'Brien JT, Ames D, Schweitzer I, Colman P, Desmond P, Tress B. Clinical and magnetic resonance imaging correlates of hypothalamic-pituitary-adrenal axis function in depression and Alzheimer's disease. Br J Psychiatry. 1996 Jun;168(6):679-87.

Osgood-Hynes DJ, Greist JH, Marks IM et al Self -administered psychotherapy for depression using a telephone-accessed computer system plus booklets: an open UK study. J Clin Psychiatry 1998 Jul; 59(7): 358-65

Owen JE, Roth DL, Stevens AB, et al Association of life events and psychological distress in family caregivers of dementia patients. Aging Ment Health. 2002 Feb;6(1):62-71.

Padberg F, Zwanzger P, Keck M, et al Repetitive Transcranial Magnetic Stimulation (rTMS) in Major Depression. Relation between Efficacy and Stimulation Intensity. Neuropsychopharmacology. 2002 Oct;27(4):638.

Palmer BW, Heaton SC, Jeste DV. Older patients with schizophrenia: Challenges in the coming decades. Psychiatric Services 1999;50 1178-1183

Parnetti L, Gaiti A, Mecocci P, et al Pharmacokinetics of IV and oral acetyl-L-carnitine in a multiple dose regimen in patients with senile dementia of Alzheimer Type. Eur. J. Clin. Pharmacol. 1992 42 (1): 89-93

Peisah C, Sachdev P, Brodaty H. Vascular dementia. International Review of Psychiatry, 1993; 5:381-395.

Penninx, B Geerlings S, Dorly J. et al Minor and Major Depression and the Risk of Death in Older Persons. Arch Gen Psych 1999 Oct; (56):889

Pennix B., Beekman A., Honig, A., et al. "Depression and Cardiac Mortality. Arch Gen Psych 2001;58: 221-227.

Perminder S, Brodaty H, JCL Looi. Vascular dementia: diagnosis, management and possible prevention. MJA 1999; 170: 81-85

Petersen RC, Smith GE, Waring SC, et al. Mild cognitive impairment: clinical characterization and outcome. Arch Neurol 1999;56: 303308

Pitzalis MV, Iacoviello M, Todarello O, Depression but not anxiety influences the autonomic control of heart rate after myocardial infarction. Am Heart J. 2001 May;141(5):765-71.

Pot AM, Deeg DJ, van Dyck R. Psychological distress of caregivers: moderator effects of caregiver resources? Patient Educ Couns. 2000 Sep;41(2):235-40.

Potkins D, Bradley S, Shrimanker J, O'Brien J, Swann A, Ballard C. End of life treatment decisions in people with dementia: carers' views and the factors which influence them. Int J Geriatr Psychiatry. 2000 Nov;15(11):1005-8.

Powers DV, Gallagher-Thompson D, Kraemer HC. Coping and depression in Alzheimer's caregivers: longitudinal evidence of stability.J Gerontol B Psychol Sci Soc Sci. 2002 May;57(3):P205-11.

Press D, Nonsteroidal drugs and Alzheimer's disease. N Engl J Med. 2002 Apr 11;346(15):1171-3.

Protas EJ, Wang CY, Harris C. Usefulness of an individualized balance and gait intervention programme based on the problem-oriented assessment of mobility in nursing home residents. Disabil Rehabil. 2001 Mar 20;23(5):192-8.

Rainer M, Mucke HA, Masching A, Haushofer M. Non-cognitive symptom profiles in dementia--experience from psychiatric services and memory clinics Psychiatr Prax. 1999 Mar;26(2):71-5.

Rantanen T, Guralnik JM, Ferrucci L, et al Coimpairments: strength and balance as predictors of severe walking disability. J Gerontol A Biol Sci Med Sci 1999 Apr;54(4):M172-6.

Rantanen T, et al. Disability, physical activity, and muscle strength in older women - The Women's Health and Aging Study. Arch Phys Med Rehabil 1999;80:130-135.

Ravnkilde B, Videbech P, Clemmensen K, et al Cognitive deficits in major depression. Scand J Psychol. 2002 Jul;43(3):239-51.

Reynolds EH. Folic acid, ageing, depression, and dementia. BMJ. 2002 Jun 22;324(7352):1512-5.

Reynolds C, Frank E, Perel J, et al Nortriptyline and Interpersonal Psychotherapy as Maintenance Therapies for Recurrent Major Depression: A Randomized Controlled Trial in Patients Older Than 59 Years, 1999; Jan 6 JAMA: (281) 39

Richards S, Hendrie H. Diagnosis, Management, and Treatment of Alzheimer Disease A Guide for the Internist. Arch Intern Med. 1999;159:789-798

Robert P. Understanding and managing behavioural symptoms in Alzheimer's disease and related dementias: focus on rivastigmine. Curr Med Res Opin. 2002;18(3):156-71.

Roberts L, Ahmed I, Hall S. Intercessory prayer for the alleviation of ill health. Cochrane Database Syst Rev. 2000;(2):CD000368

Rochon P, mith R, Aging: a global theme issue. BMJ 1996;313:1502

Rosler M, Retz W, Thome J, Riederer P. Free radicals in Alzheimer's dementia: currently available therapeutic strategies. J Neural Transm Suppl 1998;54:211-9

Ross GW, Bowen JD. The diagnosis and differential diagnosis of dementia. Med Clin North Am. 2002 May;86(3):455-76.

Rossner S Obesity in the elderly--a future matter of concern? Obes Rev. 2001 Aug;2(3):183-8.

Sable JA, Dunn LB, Zisook S. Late-life depression. How to identify its symptoms and provide effective treatment.Geriatrics. 2002 Feb;57(2):18-9, 22-3, 26 passim.

Saunders PA, Copeland JR, Dewey ME, Davidson IA, McWilliam C, Sharma V, Sullivan C. Heavy drinking as a risk factor for depression and dementia in elderly men. Findings from the Liverpool longitudinal community study. Br J Psychiatry. 1991 Aug;159:213-6.

Schaller KJ. Tai Chi Chih: an exercise option for older adults.J Gerontol Nurs. 1996 Oct;22(10):12-7.

Schlicht J, Camaione DN, Owen SV. Effect of intense strength training on standing balance, walking speed, and sit-to-stand performance in older adults. J Gerontol A Biol Sci Med Sci. 2001 May;56(5):M281

Schneider EL. Aging in the third millennium. Science 1999;283:796-79

Schoenbaum M, Un!tzer J, Sherbourne C, et al. Costeffectiveness of practice-initiated quality improvement for depression: results of a randomized controlled trial. JAMA 2001;286:11:1325-30.

Schuurman AG van den Akker M Ensinck KTJL et al Increased risk of Parkinson's disease after depression. A retrospective cohort study. Neurology 2002;58:1501-1504

Schulz R, Beach S. Caregiving as a risk factor for mortality. JAMA 1999; 282: 2215.

Seecof RL. Spirituality. J Fam Pract. 1992 Dec;35(6):617-8.

Shajahan PM, Glabus MF, Steele JD, et al Left dorso-lateral repetitive transcranial magnetic stimulation affects cortical excitability and functional connectivity, but does not impair cognition in major depression. Prog Neuropsychopharmacol Biol Psychiatry. 2002 Jun;26(5):945-54.

Sheikh JI, Yesavage JA, Brooks JO, III, Friedman LF, Gratzinger P, Hill RD, Zadeik A, Crook T: Proposed factor structure of the Geriatric Depression Scale. International Psychogeriatrics 3: 23-28, 1991.

Shigenobu K, Ikeda M, Fukuhara R, et al Reducing the burden of caring of Alzheimer's disease through the amelioration of 'delusions of theft' by drug therapy. Int J of Geriatr Psychiatry 2002; 17: 211-217.

Shua-Haim JR, Gross JS. The "co-pilot" driver syndrome. J Am Geriatr Soc 1996; 44: 815-817.

Small GW, Rabins PV, Barry PP, et al Diagnosis and treatment of Alzheimer disease and related disorders. Consensus statement of the American Association for Geriatric Psychiatry, the Alzheimer's Association, and the American Geriatrics Society. JAMA 1997 Oct 22-29;278(16):1363-71

Smith M. Mental health. Out with the old. Nurs Times. 1999 Jun 2-8;95(22):52-4

Smith RD, Widiatmoko D. The cost-effectiveness of home assessment and modification to reduce falls in the elderly. Aust N Z J Public Health 1998 Jun;22(4):436-40

Snowdon DA, Greiner LH, Mortimer JA, et al Brain infarction and the clinical expression of Alzheimer disease: the Nun Study. JAMA. 1997; 277:813-817

Solomon PR, Hirschoff A, Kelly B, et al. A 7-minute neurocognitive screening battery highly sensitive to Alzheimer's disease. Arch Neurol; 1998 55: 349355

Steffens DC, Krishnan KR, Crump C, Burke GL. Cerebrovascular disease and evolution of depressive symptoms in the cardiovascular health study. Stroke. 2002 Jun;33(6):1636-44.

St John P, Montgomery P. Are cognitively intact seniors with subjective memory loss more likely to develop dementia? Int J Geriatr Psychiatry. 2002 Sep;17(9):814-20.

Stoudemire A. Recurrence and relapse in geriatric depression: a review of risk factors and prophylactic treatment strategies. J Neuropsychiatry Clin Neurosci. 1997 Spring;9(2):208-21.

Stuck AE, Wilthert JM, Nikolaus T, et al Risk factors for functional status decline in community-living elderly people - A systematic literature review. Soc Sci Med 1999;48:445-469.

Szanto K, Gildengers A, Mulsant BH, et al Identification of suicidal ideation and prevention of suicidal behaviour in the elderly. Drugs Aging 2002;19(1):11-24

Tabet N, Feldman H. Indomethacin for the treatment of Alzheimer's disease patients. Cochrane Database Syst Rev. 2002;(2):CD003673.

Thapa PB, Gideon P, Fought RL, Ray WA Psychotropic drugs and risk of recurrent falls in ambulatory nursing home residents. Am J Epidemiol. 1995 Jul 15;142(2):202-11.

Thase ME. Treatment of severe depression. J Clin Psychiatry. 2000;61 Suppl 1:17-25

Trobe JD, Waller PF, Cook-Flanagan CA, et al. Crashes and violations among drivers with Alzheimer disease. Arch Neurol 1996; 53: 411-416.

Tsuang DW, Bird TD, Genetics of dementia. Med Clin North Am. 2002 May;86(3):591-614

Tsutsumi T, Don BM, Zaichkowsky LD, Delizonna LL. Physical fitness and psychological benefits of strength training in community dwelling older adults. Appl Human Sci. 1997 Nov;16(6):257-66.

Van Hout HP, Vernooij-Dassen MJ, Hoefnagels WH, Dementia: predictors of diagnostic accuracy and the contribution of diagnostic recommendations. J Fam Pract. 2002 Aug;51(8):693-9.

Van Someren EJ. Circadian rhythms and sleep in human aging. Chronobiol Int.
2000 May;17(3):233-43.

Vedhara K, Cox NK, Wilcock GK, et al Chronic stress in elderly carers of dementia patients and antibody response to influenza vaccination. Lancet. 1999 Feb 20;353(9153):627-31.

Vicioso BA. Dementia: when is it not Alzheimer disease?
Am J Med Sci. 2002 Aug;324(2):84-95.

Victor M. Alcoholic dementia.Can J Neurol Sci. 1994 May;21(2):88-99.

Victor M. Related Persistent altered mentation due to ethanol. Neurol Clin. 1993 Aug;11(3):639-61.

Waldemar G. Research Refines Our Understanding of the Non-Alzheimer's Dementias
The 8th International Conference on Alzheimer's Disease and Related Disorders. July 20 - 25, 2002, Stockholm, Sweden

Waldemar, G Diagnosis and management of Alzheimer's disease and other disorders associated with dementia: the role of neurologists in Europe. European Journal of Neurology, 2000 7: 133-144.

Waller PF. Renewal licensing of older drivers. Transportation in an aging society. Vol. 2. Washington, D.C.: Transportation Research Board, 1988: 72-100.

Wenger GC, Scott A, Seddon D. The experience of caring for older people with dementia in a rural area: using services. Aging Ment Health. 2002 Feb;6(1):30-8.

Wijers-Hasegawa, Y Interdisciplinary course to challenge stereotypes of old age.
March 10, 2002

The Japan Times

Wilkins K. Medications and fall-related fractures in the elderly. Health Rep.
1999 Summer;11(1):45-53(Eng); 49-58(Fre).

Wilkinson D. Clinical experience with Donepezil (Aricept) in the UK.
J Neural Transm Suppl 1998;54:311-5.

Wilson RS, de Leon CF, Barnes LL et al Participation in Cognitively Stimulating Activities and Risk of Incident Alzheimer Disease JAMA. 2002;287:742-748

Wilson RS, Barnes LL, Mendes de Leon CF, Depressive symptoms, cognitive decline, and risk of AD in older persons. Neurology. 2002 Aug 13;59(3):364-70.

Winblad B. Maintaining functional and behavioral abilities in Alzheimer disease.Alzheimer Dis Assoc Disord. 2001 Aug;15 Suppl 1:S34-40.

Witthaus E, Ott A, Barendregt JJ, et al Burden of mortality and morbidity from dementia. Alzheimer Dis Assoc Disord. 1999 Jul-Sep;13(3):176-81.

Wolf SL, Riolo L, Ouslander JG. Urge incontinence and the risk of falling in older women. J Am Geriatr Soc. 2000 Jul;48(7):847-8.

Wolf SL, Barnhart HX, Kutner NG, Reducing frailty and falls in older persons: an investigation of Tai Chi and computerized balance training. Atlanta FICSIT Group. Frailty and Injuries: Cooperative Studies of Intervention Techniques. J Am Geriatr Soc. 1996 May;44(5):489-97.

Wolfson L, Whipple R, Derby C, Balance and strength training in older adults: intervention gains and Tai Chi maintenance. J Am Geriatr Soc. 1996 May;44(5):498-506

World Health Organization, 2001. World Health Report 1997 Executive Summary. archives: 1995-2000

Yaffe K, Fox P, Newcomer R, Patient and caregiver characteristics and nursing home placement in patients with dementia. JAMA. 2002 Apr 24;287(16):2090-7

Zarit, S., Gaugler, J., & Jarrot, S. (1999). Useful services for families: Research findings and directions. Int J Geriatr Psychiatry, 14, 165-181.

Zarit S., Stephens M, Townsend A., & Greene, R. (1998). Stress reduction for family caregivers: Effects of adult day care use. J Geron: Social Sciences, 53B, S267-S277

Zarit, S., & Leitsch, S. (2001). Developing and evaluating community based intervention programs for Alzheimer's patients and their caregivers. Aging & Mental Health, 5, S84-S98.

Zimmerman SI, Girman CJ, Buie VC, et al The prevalence of osteoporosis in nursing home residents Osteoporos Int. 1999;9(2):151-7.